HESI
ADMISSION ASSESSMENT
Exam Review

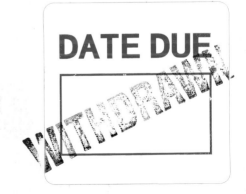

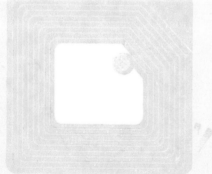

EDITION
5

HESI
ADMISSION ASSESSMENT
Exam Review

EDITOR

E. Tina Cuellar, PhD, WHNP, PMHCNS, BC
Director of Live Review
Elsevier/HESI
Houston, Texas

ELSEVIER

Elsevier
3251 Riverport Lane
St. Louis, Missouri 63043

ADMISSION ASSESSMENT *EXAM REVIEW*, FIFTH EDITION

ISBN: 978-0-323-58226-1

Previous editions copyrighted 2017, 2013, 2009, and 2004

International Standard Book Number: 978-0-323-58226-1

Senior Content Strategist: Jamie Blum
Content Development Manager: Laurie Gower
Content Development Specialist: Elizabeth McCormac
Publishing Services Manager: Shereen Jameel
Project Manager: Aparna Venkatachalam
Designer: Bridget Hoette

Printed in China

Last digit is the print number: 9 8 7 6 5 4 3 2 1

Working together to grow libraries in developing countries

www.elsevier.com • www.bookaid.org

CONTRIBUTING AUTHORS

Lisa Aberle, MSRS, RT(R)(CV)
Radiography Educator
Continuing Education
Achieve RT Media
Chatsworth, Illinois

Sandra K. Anderson, BA, LMT, ABT
Instructor
The Costa Rica School of Massage Therapy
Samara, Costa Rica

Joanna Cain, BSN, BA
President & Founder
Editorial
Auctorial Pursuits, LLC
Boulder, Colorado

John Lane, RT(R)(CT), BS, DC
Technologist
Radiography, Computed Tomography
The American Registry of Radiologic Technologists
(ARRT)
St. Louis, Missouri

PREFACE

Congratulations on purchasing the *HESI Admission Assessment Exam Review*! This study guide was developed based on the HESI Admission Assessment Exam; however, test items on the HESI Admission Assessment Exam are not specifically derived from this study guide. The content in this study guide provides an overview of the subjects tested on the Admission Assessment Exam and is designed to assist students in preparation for entrance into higher education in a variety of health-related professions. The *HESI Admission Assessment Exam Review* is written at the high school and beginning college levels and offers the basic knowledge that is necessary to be successful on the Admission Assessment Exam.

The HESI Admission Assessment exam consists of 10 different exams—8 academically oriented exams and 2 personally oriented exams. The academically oriented subjects consist of:
- Mathematics
- Reading Comprehension
- Vocabulary
- Grammar
- Biology
- Chemistry
- Anatomy and Physiology
- Physics

Chapter content in the *HESI Admission Assessment Exam Review* includes conversion tables and practice problems in the Mathematics chapter; step-by-step explanations in the Reading Comprehension and Grammar chapters; a substantial list of words used in health professions in the Vocabulary chapter; rationales and sample questions in the Biology and Chemistry chapters; helpful terminology in the Anatomy and Physiology chapter; and sample problems in the Physics chapter. Also included throughout the exam review are "HESI Hint" boxes, which are designed to offer students a suggestion, an example, or a reminder pertaining to a specific topic.

The personally oriented exams consist of a Learning Style assessment and a Personality Profile. These exams are intended to offer students insights into their study habits, learning preferences, and dispositions relating to academic achievement. Students generally like to take these personally oriented exams for the purpose of personal insight and discussion. Because each of these exams takes only approximately 15 minutes to complete, the school may include them in their administration of the Admission Assessment Exam.

Schools can choose to administer any one, or all, of these exams provided by the Admission Assessment. For example, programs that do not require biology, chemistry, anatomy and physiology, or physics for entry would not administer those specific Admission Assessment science-oriented exams.

The HESI Admission Assessment Exam has been used by colleges, universities, and health-related institutions as part of the selection and placement process for applicants and newly admitted students for approximately 10 years.

Study Hints

It is always a good idea to prepare for any exam. When you begin to study for the Admission Assessment Exam, make sure you allocate adequate time and do not feel rushed. Set up a schedule that provides an hour or two each day to review material in the *HESI Admission Assessment Exam Review*. Mark the time you set aside on a calendar to remind yourself when to study each day. Before you begin, take the 25-question Pretest at the beginning of the text to help you initially assess your strengths and weaknesses of the content. For each section in the *HESI Admission Assessment Exam Review*, review the material that is relevant to your particular field of the health care professions. Complete the review questions at the end of each chapter, then complete the 50-question Posttest at the end of the text. This Posttest gives you additional practice in the text's subject areas using a more comprehensive approach. The

Posttest will help you to assess your readiness for the exam. Once you have completed your review and self-assessment of topics in the study guide, more test-taking practice is available on the text's corresponding Evolve site (http://www.elsevier.com/HESI/A2Review) with two comprehensive 82-question Practice Exams on the various subject areas that will help you prepare for the Admissions Assessment Exam. If you are having trouble with the review questions or the Practice Exams for a particular section, review that content in the *HESI Admission Assessment Exam Review* study guide again. It may also be helpful to go back to your textbook and class notes for additional review.

Test-Taking Hints

1. Read each question carefully and completely. Make sure you understand what the question is asking.
2. Identify the key words or phrases in the question. These words or phrases will provide critical information about how to answer the question.
3. Rephrase the question in your words.
   A. Ask yourself, "What is the question really asking?"
   B. Eliminate nonessential information from the question.
   C. Sometimes writers use terminology that may be unfamiliar to you. Do not be confused by a new writing style.
4. Rule out options (if they are presented).
   A. Read all of the responses completely.
   B. Rule out any options that are clearly incorrect.
   C. Mentally mark through incorrect options in your head.
   D. Differentiate between the remaining options, considering your knowledge of the subject.
5. Computer tests do not allow an option for skipping questions and returning to them later. Practice answering every question as it appears.

Do not second-guess yourself. TRUST YOUR ANSWERS.

CONTENTS

1. A pair of six-sided dice is rolled one time. What is the probability that the number 5 will appear?
   A. 1/12
   B. 1/6
   C. 1/4
   D. 1/3

2. The nurse's notation describes the patient as "febrile." Based on this information, which statement is true?
   A. The patient is confused.
   B. The patient had a seizure.
   C. The patient feels weak.
   D. The patient has a fever.

3. In the hierarchic system of classification, which is the largest?
   A. Kingdom
   B. Class
   C. Genus
   D. Species

4. Which structure is part of the respiratory system?
   A. Esophagus
   B. Trachea
   C. Pancreas
   D. Spleen

5. Write the following quantity, 1 millimeter (mm), in powers of tens: _____

6. The product of y and -25 is -100; find the value of y.
   A. 4
   B. -2500
   C. -4
   D. 2500

Use the passage below to answer questions 7-9.

Penicillin

Antibiotics are among the most commonly prescribed drugs today. Before the discovery of the first antibiotic, there was no effective treatment for bacterial infections such as pneumonia. Until antibiotics were available, even a tiny cut on the surface of the skin could result in a potentially grave infection.

The world's first true antibiotic was discovered by a professor of bacteriology named Alexander Fleming. In 1928, Fleming was performing experiments with staphylococcal bacteria. Fleming noticed that the bacteria in one of his Petri dishes was dying. Unlike the other samples, this dish had become contaminated by mold spores. Fleming was able to identify the mold as a member of the *Penicillium* genus.

When Fleming grew this mold in a pure culture, he found that it produced a substance that was effective against all Gram-positive pathogens. He would eventually name this "mold juice" penicillin. Fleming admitted that his discovery was purely accidental, but his groundbreaking work in developing the first antibiotic revolutionized medicine and saved millions of lives.

7. Which is the author's primary purpose in writing this essay?
   A. To entertain the reader with stories about a famous inventor.
   B. To explain how antibiotics are able to destroy bacteria.
   C. To inform the reader about how penicillin was discovered.
   D. To analyze the difference between types of bacteria.

8. According to the passage, which statement is **false**?
   A. Penicillin is effective against Gram-positive pathogens.
   B. One of Fleming's Petri dishes became contaminated with bacteria.
   C. Fleming discovered penicillin by accident.
   D. Fleming discovered the first antibiotic.

9. What is the meaning of the word *grave* in the first paragraph?
   A. Very serious
   B. Incurable
   C. Highly contagious
   D. Deadly

10. A paramedic treats a patient who has a deep cut in the skin caused by broken glass. Which term best describes this injury?
    A. Incision
    B. Laceration
    C. Puncture
    D. Abrasion

11. Which word in the following sentence is a verb?
    Roy was afraid he would not be able to finish the race.
    A. was
    B. afraid
    C. able
    D. race

12. Twelve (12) more than a number is five (5). What is the number?
    A. −7
    B. 7
    C. −17
    D. 17

13. Select the best word for the blank in the following sentence.
    I must remember to _____ my book to class today.
    A. Bring
    B. Take
    C. Brought
    D. Took

14. Which subatomic particles contain a positive charge?
    A. Protons and electrons
    B. Protons only
    C. Protons and neutrons
    D. Neutrons and electrons

15. After observing an event, you develop an explanation. This explanation is tested by performing a repeatable procedure. What is this procedure called?
    A. Hypothesis
    B. Experiment
    C. Conclusion
    D. Theory

16. Which word in the following sentence is the direct object?
    Tom's dad gave him a bicycle for his birthday.
    A. dad
    B. him
    C. bicycle
    D. birthday

17. Which property of water explains why the oceans are helpful in stabilizing the climate?
    A. Water molecules spread apart in freezing temperatures.
    B. Water has strong cohesive and adhesive properties.
    C. Water can act as both an acid and a base.
    D. Water has a relatively high specific heat value.

18. Select the meaning of the underlined word in the sentence.
    She felt dizzy and had difficulty ambulating.
    A. Walking
    B. Balancing
    C. Seeing
    D. Standing

19. Calcium is located in group IIA on the periodic table. Which is the charge on a calcium ion?
    A. −1
    B. +1
    C. −2
    D. +2

20. Which is the unit for measuring the amount of force applied to an object?
    A. Joules
    B. Hertz
    C. Newtons
    D. Watts

21. Which mineral is necessary for muscle contraction?
    A. Chloride
    B. Sodium
    C. Calcium
    D. Magnesium

22. Which biological molecules are composed of amino acids?
    A. Carbohydrates
    B. Lipids
    C. Proteins
    D. Nucleic acids

23. Which is the correct coefficient for water (H_2O) when the following equation is balanced?
    $$2C_2H_6 + 7O_2 \rightarrow 4CO_2 + \_H_2O$$
    A. 3 parts H_2O
    B. 6 parts H_2O
    C. 9 parts H_2O
    D. 14 parts H_2O

24. A tissue examined under the microscope is from the internal surface of stomach, has layers of flat cells, and is without blood vessels. Which type of tissue is this?
    A. Epithelial
    B. Connective
    C. Muscle
    D. Nervous

25. Which physical quantity has both a magnitude and a direction?
    A. Energy
    B. Time
    C. Velocity
    D. Distance

ANSWERS TO PRETEST

1. D—There is 1 out of 6 chances on 1 die. When rolling a pair of dice, there are 12 chances in 36 possible outcomes. A 12-to-36 chance is equal to 1 out of 3.
2. D
3. A
4. B
5. 10^{-3} mm
6. A—Divide: $-100 \div -25 = 4$
7. C
8. B
9. A
10. B
11. A
12. A—Add -12 to 5. The solution is -7.
13. B—In this sentence, the action is away from the speaker, who will carry the book from a near place (where the speaker is) to a far place (the classroom). Therefore, the best word is "take."
14. B
15. B
16. C—The direct object is the word that is directly affected by the action of the verb. In this sentence, the noun "bicycle" receives the action of the verb "gave."
17. D
18. A
19. D
20. C
21. C
22. C
23. B
24. A
25. C

HESI
ADMISSION ASSESSMENT
Exam Review

MATHEMATICS

Members of the health professions use math every day to calculate medication dosages, radiation limits, nutritional needs, mental status, intravenous drip rates, intake and output, and a host of other requirements related to their clients. Safe and effective care is the goal of all who work in health professions. Therefore, it is essential that students entering the health professions understand and make calculations using whole numbers, fractions, decimals, and percentages.

The purpose of this chapter is to review the addition, subtraction, multiplication, and division of whole numbers, fractions, decimals, and percentages. Basic algebra skills will also be reviewed, such as evaluating expressions, and solving for a specific variable. Mastery of these basic mathematic functions is an integral step toward a career in the health professions.

CHAPTER OUTLINE

Basic Addition and Subtraction
Basic Multiplication (Whole Numbers)
Basic Division (Whole Numbers)
Decimals
Fractions

Multiplication of Fractions
Division of Fractions
Changing Fractions to Decimals
Changing Decimals to Fractions
Ratios and Proportions
Percentages

12-hour Clock versus Military Time
Algebra
Helpful Information to Memorize
Answers to Sample Problems

KEY TERMS

Common Denominator
Constant
Denominator
Digit
Dividend
Divisor
Exponent
Expression

Factor
Fraction Bar
Improper Fraction
Least Common Denominator
Numerator
Percent
Place Value
Product

Proper Fraction
Proportion
Quotient
Ratio
Reciprocals
Remainder
Terminating Decimal
Variable

Basic Addition and Subtraction

Digit: Any number 1 through 9 and 0 (e.g., the number 7 is a digit)
Place Value: The value of the position of a digit in a number (e.g., in the number 321, the number 2 is in the "tens" position)

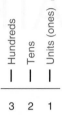

Hundreds	Tens	Units (ones)
3	2	1

HESI Hint

1 ten = 10 ones
1 hundred = 100 ones
1 thousand = 1000 ones

Basic Addition

Example 1

382 + 212

$$\begin{array}{r} 382 \\ + \ 212 \\ \hline 594 \end{array}$$

Steps

1. Line up the **digits** according to **place value.**
2. Add the digits starting from right to left.
   - Ones: 2 + 2 = 4
   - Tens: 8 + 1 = 9
   - Hundreds: 3 + 2 = 5

Addition with Regrouping

HESI Hint

To solve an addition problem, it may be necessary to regroup by moving, or carrying over, an extra digit from one place value column to the next.

Example 2

748 + 523

$$\begin{array}{r} \overset{1}{7}48 \\ + \ 523 \\ \hline 1{,}271 \end{array}$$

Steps

1. Line up the digits according to place value.
2. Add:
   - Ones: 8 + 3 = 11
   - Carry the 1 to the tens place, which is one place to the left.
   - Tens: 1 + 4 + 2 = 7
   - Hundreds: 7 + 5 = 12

Basic Subtraction

Subtraction provides the difference between two numbers.

HESI Hint

It may be easier to solve a subtraction problem by first rewriting it vertically.

Example 1

3,884 − 1,671

$$
\begin{array}{r}
3,884 \\
- 1,671 \\
\hline
2,213
\end{array}
$$

Steps

1. Line up the digits according to place value.
2. Subtract:
   - Ones: 4 − 1 = 3
   - Tens: 8 − 7 = 1
   - Hundreds: 8 − 6 = 2
   - Thousands: 3 − 1 = 2

Subtraction with Regrouping

HESI Hint

Remember, if the number to subtract is not a positive number, you must borrow or regroup from one place value to a lower place value.

Example 1

862 − 57

$$
\begin{array}{r}
{\scriptstyle 5\ 12} \\
8\,\cancel{6}\,\cancel{2} \\
-5\ 7 \\
\hline
8\ 0\ 5
\end{array}
$$

Steps

1. Align the digits according to place value.
2. Subtract:
   - Ones: 12 − 7 = 5
   - Tens: 5 − 5 = 0
   - Hundreds: 8 − 0 = 8

Add or subtract each of the following problems as indicated.

1. 1,283 + 188 =
2. 273 + 47 =
3. 1,644 + 357 =
4. 73 + 211 + 22 =
5. 382 − 150 =
6. 246 − 47 =
7. 568 − 170 =
8. 17,444 − 923 =
9. Sam walks 2 blocks to Stacey's house. They both walk 5 blocks to the park. How far has Sam walked?
10. Lisa buys 12 eggs from the store so she can make pancakes. The pancake recipe calls for 3 eggs. How many eggs will Lisa have left after making the pancakes?

Basic Multiplication (Whole Numbers)

The process of multiplication is essentially repeated addition.

Product: The answer to a multiplication problem.

HESI Hint

Remember, the zero is used as a placeholder to keep the problem aligned. If you do not skip a space, the answer will be incorrect. Below is an example of a well-aligned problem.

$$
\begin{array}{r}
24571 \\
\times\ 1233 \\
\hline
73{,}713 \\
737{,}130 \\
4{,}914{,}200 \\
+\ 24{,}571{,}000 \\
\hline
30{,}296{,}043 \\
\end{array}
\begin{array}{l}
\\
\\
\rightarrow \text{Ones} \\
\rightarrow \text{Tens} \\
\rightarrow \text{Hundreds} \\
\rightarrow \text{Thousands} \\
\end{array}
$$

Example 1

18×4

$$
\begin{array}{r}
\overset{3}{1}8 \\
\times\ 4 \\
\hline
72 \\
\end{array}
$$

Steps

1. Multiply one digit at a time.
2. Multiply 4×18.
   - Ones: $4 \times 8 = 32$
   Carry the 1 to the tens place, and write the 2 in the ones place.
   - Tens: $4 \times 1 = 4 + 3 = 7$

Example 2

713×24

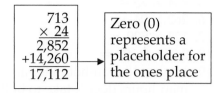

```
     713
  ×   24
   2,852
 +14,260
  17,112
```

Zero (0) represents a placeholder for the ones place

Steps

1. Multiply 713×24.
   - $4 \times 3 = 12$
   - $4 \times 1 = 4 + 1 = 5$
   - $4 \times 7 = 28$
2. Multiply 713×2 (remember to line up the ones digit with the 4 by using zero as a placeholder).
   - $2 \times 3 = 6$
   - $2 \times 1 = 2$
   - $2 \times 7 = 14$
3. Add the two products together.
   - $2,852 + 14,260 = 17,112$ (the final **product**)

Example 3

411×242

```
     411
  ×  242
     822
  16,440
 + 82,200
  99,462
```

Steps

1. Multiply 411×2.
   - $2 \times 1 = 2$
   - $2 \times 1 = 2$
   - $2 \times 4 = 8$
2. Multiply 411×4.
   - $4 \times 1 = 4$ (remember to use a zero for a placeholder)
   - $4 \times 1 = 4$
   - $4 \times 4 = 16$
3. Multiply 411×2.
   - $2 \times 1 = 2$
   - $2 \times 1 = 2$
   - $2 \times 4 = 8$
4. Add the three products together.
   - $822 + 16,440 + 82,200 = 99,462$ (the final **product**)

SAMPLE PROBLEMS

Multiply each of the following problems as indicated.

1. $246 \times 4 =$
2. $689 \times 2 =$

3. $821 \times 22 =$
4. $529 \times 47 =$
5. $954 \times 75 =$
6. $262 \times 94 =$
7. $123 \times 529 =$
8. $2{,}943 \times 293 =$
9. It takes 18 man-hours for an automobile factory to build a car. How many man-hours does it take to build 92 cars?
10. A bakery sells boxes of donuts with 13 donuts in each box. If the bakery sells 52 boxes of donuts, how many total donuts were sold?

Basic Division (Whole Numbers)

Dividend: The number being divided.
Divisor: The number by which the dividend is divided.
Quotient: The answer to a division problem.
Remainder: The portion of the dividend that is not evenly divisible by the divisor.

HESI Hint

$$\begin{array}{r} 9 \\ 5\overline{)45} \end{array}$$

The 45 represents the **dividend** (the number being divided), the 5 represents the **divisor** (the number by which the dividend is divided), and the 9 represents the **quotient** (the answer to the division problem). It is best not to leave a division problem with a **remainder,** but to end it as a fraction or decimal instead. To make the problem into a decimal, add a decimal point and zeros at the end of the dividend and continue. If a remainder continues to occur, round to the hundredths place.

Example

$233.547 \rightarrow 233.55$ (the 7 rounds the 4 to a 5)

Example 1

$42 \div 7$

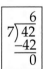

Steps

1. Set up the problem.
2. Use a series of multiplication and subtraction problems to solve a division problem.
3. $7 \times ? = 42$
   - Multiply: $7 \times 6 = 42$
   - Subtract: $42 - 42 = 0$
   - The quotient (or answer) is 6.

Example 2

$464 \div 4$

$$
\begin{array}{r}
116 \\
4\overline{)464} \\
-4\downarrow\downarrow \\
\overline{06}\downarrow \\
-4\downarrow \\
\overline{24} \\
-24 \\
\overline{0}
\end{array}
$$

Steps

1. Set up the problem.
2. Begin with the hundreds place.
   - $4 \times ? = 4$. We know $4 \times 1 = 4$; therefore, place the 1 (quotient) above the 4 in the hundreds place (dividend). Place the other 4 under the hundreds place and subtract: $4 - 4 = 0$.
   - Bring down the next number, which is 6; $4 \times ? = 6$. There is no number that can be multiplied by 4 that will equal 6 exactly, so try to get as close as possible without going over 6. Use $4 \times 1 = 4$ and set it up just like the last subtraction problem: $6 - 4 = 2$.
   - Bring down the 4 from the dividend, which results in the number 24 (the 2 came from the remainder of $6 - 4 = 2$).
   - $4 \times ? = 24$; $? = 6$. The two becomes the next number in the quotient. $24 - 24 = 0$. There is no remainder left.
   - The quotient (or answer) is 116.

Example 3

$163 \div 5$

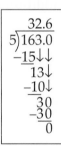

$$
\begin{array}{r}
32.6 \\
5\overline{)163.0} \\
-15\downarrow\downarrow \\
\overline{13}\downarrow \\
-10\downarrow \\
\overline{30} \\
-30 \\
\overline{0}
\end{array}
$$

Steps

1. Set up the problem.
2. The 5 (divisor) does not divide into 1 but does divide into 16.
3. $5 \times 3 = 15$. Write the 3 in the quotient. (It is written above the 6 in 16 because that is the last digit in the number.)
   - $5 \times 3 = 15$
   - $16 - 15 = 1$
4. Bring the 3 down. Combine the 1 (remainder from $16 - 15$) and 3 to create 13.
5. The 5 does not divide evenly into 13; therefore, try to get close without going over.
   - $5 \times 2 = 10$
   - $13 - 10 = 3$

6. There is a remainder of 3, but there is no number left in the dividend. Add a decimal point and zeros and continue to divide.
7. The quotient (or answer) is 32.6 (thirty-two and six tenths).

SAMPLE PROBLEMS

Divide in each of the following problems as indicated.
1. $135 \div 9 =$
2. $8{,}400 \div 4 =$
3. $3{,}732 \div 2 =$
4. $357 \div 17 =$
5. $4{,}725 \div 9 =$
6. $2{,}925 \div 3 =$
7. $787 \div 8 =$
8. $6{,}281 \div 5 =$
9. There are 72 bottles of water for a soccer team with 16 players. If each player receives the same amount of water, how many bottles of water can each player have?
10. Tim is driving 270 miles to visit his parents. Tim's car can travel 18 miles on 1 gallon of gas. How many gallons of gas does Tim need to make it to his parents' house?

Decimals

A decimal pertains to tenths or to the number 10.

Place value: Regarding decimals, numbers to the right of the decimal point have different terms from the whole numbers to the left of the decimal point. Each digit in a number occupies a position called a **place value.**

Addition and Subtraction of Decimals

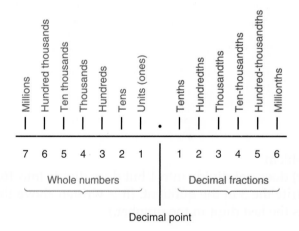

Millions	Hundred thousands	Ten thousands	Thousands	Hundreds	Tens	Units (ones)		Tenths	Hundredths	Thousandths	Ten-thousandths	Hundred-thousandths	Millionths
7	6	5	4	3	2	1		1	2	3	4	5	6

Whole numbers — Decimal fractions

Decimal point

Example 1

1.3 + 7.2

$$\begin{array}{r} 1.3 \\ + \ 7.2 \\ \hline 8.5 \end{array}$$

Steps

1. Align the decimal points.
2. Add the tenths together: 3 + 2 = 5
3. Add the ones together: 1 + 7 = 8
4. Final answer: 8.5 (eight and five tenths).

Example 2

6 + 22.13

$$\begin{array}{r} 22.13 \\ + \ 6.00 \\ \hline 28.13 \end{array}$$

Steps

1. Align the decimal points.
   - It might be difficult to align the 6 because it does not have a decimal point.
   - Remember that after the ones place, there is a decimal point. To help with organization, add zeros (placeholders). **Example:** 6 = 6.00
2. Add the hundredths: 3 + 0 = 3
3. Add the tenths: 1 + 0 = 1
4. Add the ones: 2 + 6 = 8
5. Add the tens: 2 + 0 = 2
6. Final answer: 28.13 (twenty-eight and thirteen hundredths).

Example 3

9.46 − 7.34

$$\begin{array}{r} 9.46 \\ - \ 7.34 \\ \hline 2.12 \end{array}$$

Steps

1. Align the decimal points.
2. Subtract the hundredths: 6 − 4 = 2
3. Subtract the tenths: 4 − 3 = 1
4. Subtract the ones: 9 − 7 = 2
5. Final answer: 2.12 (two and twelve hundredths).

Example 4

22 − 7.99

$$
\begin{array}{r}
\overset{\scriptstyle 1\ \ \ 9\ 10}{2\cancel{2}.\cancel{0}\cancel{0}} \\
-7.99 \\
\hline
14.01
\end{array}
$$

Steps

1. Align the decimal points.
2. Because 22 is a whole number, add a decimal point and zeros.
3. 0.00 − 0.99 cannot be subtracted; therefore, 1 must be borrowed from the 22 and regrouped.
4. The ones become 1, the tenths become 9, and the hundredths become 10.
5. Subtract the hundredths: 10 − 9 = 1
6. Subtract the tenths: 9 − 9 = 0
7. Subtract the ones: 21 − 7 = 14
   - 1 was borrowed from the tens in order to subtract the 7.
8. Final answer: 14.01 (fourteen and one hundredth).

SAMPLE PROBLEMS

Solve each of the following decimal problems as indicated.
1. 2.7 + 8.44 =
2. 7.125 + 38.65 =
3. 127.2 + 83 =
4. 43 + 9.57 =
5. 4.6 + 3.66 + 11 =
6. 22 − 14.18 =
7. 67.74 − 9.83 =
8. 17.56 − 9.88 =
9. Robin used the company car for 3 business trips. She traveled 3.2 miles on Monday, 4.75 miles on Wednesday, and 7.3 miles on Friday. How many total miles did Robin travel for the week?
10. A dressmaker needs 4.25 yards of fabric to make a blue dress, but only 2.5 yards of blue fabric are left in stock. How many additional yards of fabric does the dressmaker need to complete the dress?

Multiplication of Decimals

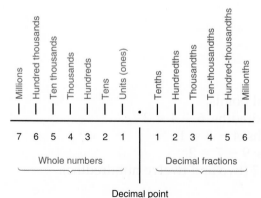

Example 1

81.2 + 4.2

$\begin{array}{r} 81.2 \\ \times\ 4.2 \\ \hline 1624 \\ +\ 32480 \\ \hline 341.04 \end{array}$	1 decimal place + 1 decimal place ————————— 2 decimal places Move the decimal point two places to the left in the final product.

Steps

1. Multiply 812 × 42 (do not worry about the decimal point until the final product has been calculated).
2. Starting from the right, count the decimal places in both numbers and add together (two decimal places).
3. Move to the left two places, and then place the decimal point.

Example 2

0.002 + 3.4

$\begin{array}{r} 0.002 \\ \times\quad 3.4 \\ \hline 0008 \\ +\ 00060 \\ \hline 0.0068 \end{array}$	3 decimal places + 1 decimal place ————————— 4 decimal places Move four places to the left.

Steps

1. Multiply 2 × 34.
2. Starting from the right, count the decimal places in both numbers and add together (four decimal places).
3. Move to the left four places, and then place the decimal.

Example 3

8.23 × 3

$\begin{array}{r} 8.23 \\ \times\quad 3 \\ \hline 24.69 \end{array}$	2 decimal places + 0 decimal places ————————— 2 decimal places Move two places to the left.

Steps

1. Multiply 823 × 3.
2. Starting from the right, count the decimal places in both numbers and add together (two decimal places).
3. Move to the left two places, and then place the decimal point.

SAMPLE PROBLEMS

Multiply the decimals in the following problems as indicated.
1. $0.012 \times 3.27 =$
2. $22.79 \times 6 =$
3. $4.04 \times 6.1 =$
4. $321.1 \times 18 =$
5. $0.9112 \times 8.13 =$
6. $21.2 \times 7 =$
7. $0.009 \times 45.2 =$
8. $245.24 \times .003 =$
9. Tina's water bottle holds 24.6 ounces of liquid. If Tina drinks 2.5 bottles of water, how much water has she drunk?
10. Dennis walks 1.2 miles to the store to buy groceries. He walks another 1.2 miles to bring the groceries home. How many miles does Dennis have to walk to complete 2 grocery trips?

Division of Decimals

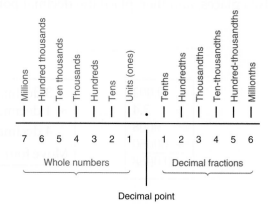

HESI Hint

The number 25 is a whole number. Though this number could be written 25.0, decimals are usually not displayed after a whole number.

Example 1

$48 \div 2.5$

```
              19.2
      2.5 ) 48.0.0
           −25 ↓↓
            230↓
           −225↓
             50
            −50
              0
```

Steps

1. Set up the division problem.
2. Move the decimal point in 2.5 one place to the right, making it a whole number.

3. What is done to one side must be done to the other side. Move the decimal point one place to the right in 48, making it 480, and then bring the decimal point up into the quotient.
4. Divide normally.
   - $25 \times 1 = 25$
   - Subtract: $48 - 25 = 23$
   - Bring down the zero to make 230.
   - $25 \times 9 = 225$. This is as close to 230 as possible without going over.
   - Subtract: $230 - 225 = 5$
   - Add a zero to the dividend and bring it down to the 5, making it 50.
   - $25 \times 2 = 50$
   - $50 - 50 = 0$
5. The quotient is 19.2.

Example 2

$2.468 \div 0.2$

Steps

1. Set up the division problem.
2. Move the decimal point in 0.2 over one place to the right, making it a whole number. 0.2 is now 2.
3. Move the same number of spaces in the dividend. 2.468 is now 24.68.
4. Bring the decimal point up to the quotient in the new position.
5. Divide normally.

Example 3

$0.854 \div 0.05$

$$\begin{array}{r} 17.08 \\ 0.05\overline{)0.85.40} \\ -5\downarrow\downarrow\downarrow \\ 35\downarrow\downarrow \\ -35\downarrow\downarrow \\ 040 \\ -40 \\ \hline 0 \end{array}$$

Steps

1. Set up the division problem.
2. Move the decimal point in the divisor until it is a whole number. 0.05 is now 5.
3. Move the decimal point in the dividend the same number of spaces as was moved in the divisor. 0.854 is now 85.4.
4. Divide normally.

SAMPLE PROBLEMS

Divide the decimals in the following problems as indicated.
1. $36 \div 0.8 =$
2. $54 \div 0.3 =$
3. $65.6 \div 0.8 =$
4. $43.54 \div 0.7 =$

5. $5.202 \div 0.45 =$
6. $912 \div 0.2 =$
7. $0.052 \div 0.8 =$
8. $0.624 \div 0.26 =$
9. Dan's pie crust recipe calls for 1.25 ounces of canola oil per crust. How many pie crusts can Dan make if he has 10 ounces of canola oil?
10. A carpenter is cutting a board to make shelves for a bookcase. The board is 2.44 meters long and 0.3 meters wide. Each shelf will be 0.61 meters long and 0.3 meters wide. How many shelves will the bookcase have?

Fractions

In mathematics, a fraction is a way to express a part in relation to the total.
Numerator: The top number in a fraction.
Denominator: The bottom number in a fraction.
Fraction Bar: The line between the numerator and denominator. The bar is another symbol for division.
Factor: A number that divides evenly into another number.
Least Common Denominator (LCD): The smallest multiple that two numbers share.
Improper Fraction: A fraction where the numerator is larger than the denominator.
Proper Fraction: A fraction where the denominator is larger than the numerator.
Common Denominator: Two or more fractions having the same denominator.
Reciprocals: Pairs of numbers that equal 1 when multiplied together.
Terminating Decimal: A decimal that is not continuous.

HESI Hint

- The **numerator** is the top number of the fraction. It represents the part or pieces.
- The **denominator** is the bottom number of the fraction. It represents the total or whole amount.
- The fraction bar is the line that separates the numerator and the denominator.

$$\frac{\text{Numerator (part)}}{\text{Denominator (whole)}} \text{Fraction bar}$$

Reducing Fractions Using the Greatest Common Factor

A **factor** is a number that divides evenly into another number.
   Factors of 12:
- $1 \times 12 = 12$
- $2 \times 6 = 12$
- $3 \times 4 = 12$

12 {1, 2, 3, 4, 6, 12}: Listing the factors helps determine the greatest common factor between two or more numbers.

$$\frac{1}{2} = \frac{2}{4}, \frac{3}{6}, \frac{4}{8}, \frac{5}{10}, \frac{6}{12}, \frac{7}{14}, \frac{8}{16}, \frac{9}{18}, \frac{10}{20}$$

All represent one-half.
   Reducing fractions can also be called reducing a fraction to its lowest terms or simplest form. A fraction is reduced to the lowest terms by finding an equivalent fraction in which the numerator and denominator are as small as possible. You may need to reduce fractions to work with them in an equation or

for solving a problem. That means that there is no number, except 1, that can be divided evenly into both the numerator and the denominator.

$$1 = \frac{1}{1}, \frac{2}{2}, \frac{3}{3}, \frac{4}{4}, \frac{5}{5}, \frac{6}{6}, \frac{7}{7}, \frac{8}{8}, \frac{9}{9}, \frac{10}{10}$$

Example 1

Reduce $\dfrac{4}{24}$

Factors of 4 and 24:
4 {1, 2, 4}
24 {1, 2, 4, 6, 8, 12}
The greatest common factor is 4; therefore, divide the numerator and denominator by 4.

$$\frac{4}{24} \div \frac{4}{4} = \frac{1}{6}$$

Example 2

Reduce $\dfrac{12}{20}$

Factors of 12 and 20:
12 {1, 2, 3, **4**, 6, 12}
20 {1, 2, **4**, 5, 10, 20}
The greatest common factor is 4 (they do have 1 and 2 in common, but the greatest factor is best).

$$\frac{12}{20} \div \frac{4}{4} = \frac{3}{5}$$

Least Common Denominator

The LCD is the smallest multiple that two numbers share. Determining the LCD is an essential step in the addition, subtraction, and ordering of fractions.

Example 1

Find the LCD for $\dfrac{3}{4}$ and $\dfrac{7}{9}$

Steps

1. List the multiples (multiplication tables) of each denominator.
   - 4: $4 \times 1 = 4, 4 \times 2 = 8, 4 \times 3 = 12, 4 \times 4 = 16, 4 \times 5 = 20, 4 \times 6 = 24, 4 \times 7 = 28, 4 \times 8 = 32, 4 \times 9 = 36, 4 \times 10 = 40$
   - 4 {4, 8, 12, 16, 20, 24, 28, 32, 36, 40}—this will be the standard form throughout for listing multiples.
   - 9 {9, 18, 27, 36, 45, 54, 63, 72, 81, 90}
2. Compare each for the least common multiple.
   - 4 {4, 8, 12, 16, 20, 24, 28, 32, **36**, 40}
   - 9 {9, 18, 27, **36**, 45, 54, 63, 72, 81, 90}
3. The LCD between 4 and 9 is 36 ($4 \times 9 = 36$ and $9 \times 4 = 36$).

Example 2

Find the LCD for $\dfrac{1}{15}$ and $\dfrac{2}{3}$.

Steps

1. List the multiples of each denominator, and find the common multiples.
   - 15 {**15**, 30, 45, 60, 75, 90, 105, 120, 135, 150}
   - 3 {3, 6, 9, 12, **15**, 18, 21, 24, 27, 30}
2. The LCD between 15 and 3 is 15 (15 × 1 = 15 and 3 × 5 is 15).

Changing Improper Fractions into Mixed Numbers

An **improper fraction** occurs when the numerator is larger than the denominator. An improper fraction should be reduced and made into a mixed number.

Example

$$\frac{17}{5} \to 5\overline{)\begin{array}{r} 3 \\ 17 \\ \underline{15} \\ 2 \end{array}} \to 3\frac{2}{5}$$

Steps

1. Turn an improper fraction into a mixed number through division. (The top number [numerator] goes in the box [17]; the bottom number [denominator] stays out [5].)
2. The 3 becomes the whole number.
3. The remainder (2) becomes the numerator.
4. The denominator stays the same.

Changing Mixed Numbers into Improper Fractions

A mixed number has a whole number and fraction combined.

Example

$$5\frac{2}{3} \to 5\frac{+2}{3} = (5 \times 3) + 2 = 17 \to \frac{17}{3}$$

Steps

1. To make a mixed number into an improper fraction, multiply the denominator (3) and whole number (5) together, then add the numerator (2).
2. Place this new numerator (17) over the denominator (3), which stays the same in the mixed number.

Addition of Fractions

Addition with Common Denominators

Example

$$\frac{1}{9} + \frac{7}{9} = \frac{8}{9}$$

Steps

1. Add the numerators together: 1 + 7 = 8.
2. The denominator (9) stays the same. This makes it a **common denominator.**
3. Answer: $\frac{8}{9}$ (eight ninths).

Addition with Unlike Denominators

Example

$$\frac{1}{3} + \frac{4}{9}$$

$$\frac{1 \times 3}{3 \times 3} = \frac{3}{9}$$

$$\frac{4 \times 1}{9 \times 1} = \frac{4}{9}$$

$$\frac{3}{9} + \frac{4}{9} = \frac{7}{9}$$

Steps

1. Find the LCD by listing the multiples of each denominator.
   - 3 {3, 6, **9**, 12, 15}
   - 9 {**9**, 27, 36, 45}
   - The LCD is 9.
2. If the denominator is changed, the numerator must also be changed by the same number. Do this by multiplying the numerator and denominator by the same number.

$$\frac{1 \times 3}{3 \times 3} = \frac{3}{9}$$

3. Because the denominator of the second fraction is 9, no change is necessary.
4. Add the numerators together, and keep the common denominator.
5. Reduce the fraction if necessary.

Addition of Mixed Numbers

Example

$$2\frac{1}{3} + 3\frac{11}{15}$$

$$2\frac{1 \times 5}{3 \times 5} = 2\frac{5}{15}$$

$$3\frac{11 \times 1}{15 \times 1} = 3\frac{11}{15}$$

$$2\frac{5}{15} + 3\frac{11}{15} = 5\frac{16}{15} = 6\frac{1}{15}$$

Steps

1. Find the LCD of 3 and 15 by listing the multiples of each.
   - 3 (3, 6, 9, 12, **15**)
   - 15 (**15**, 30, 45)
2. Calculate the new numerator of each fraction to correspond to the changed denominator.

3. Add the whole numbers together, and then add the numerators together. Keep the common denominator 15.
4. The numerator is larger than the denominator (improper); change the answer to a mixed number (review vocabulary if necessary).

SAMPLE PROBLEMS

Add the fractions in the following problems as indicated (remember to reduce the fraction as needed).

1. $\dfrac{2}{10} + \dfrac{5}{10} =$

2. $\dfrac{4}{18} + \dfrac{11}{18} =$

3. $\dfrac{4}{6} + \dfrac{7}{6} =$

4. $\dfrac{5}{8} + \dfrac{1}{16} =$

5. $\dfrac{7}{9} + \dfrac{6}{11} =$

6. $6\dfrac{2}{3} + 4\dfrac{5}{12} =$

7. $2\dfrac{2}{7} + 3\dfrac{2}{9} =$

8. $5\dfrac{1}{6} + 3\dfrac{2}{18} =$

9. Ray is driving Tom to the movies. Tom lives 2½ miles from Ray's house. The movie theatre is 1¾ miles from Tom's house. How many miles must Ray drive to pick up Tom and drive to the theatre?
10. The Warrens are installing a privacy fence along two sides of their property. The length of one side is 85⅓ feet. The length of the other side is 62⅚ feet. How many feet of fencing will the Warrens install?

Subtraction of Fractions

Subtracting Fractions with Common Denominators

Example

$$\frac{5}{6} - \frac{1}{6} = \frac{4}{6} = \frac{2}{3}$$

Steps

1. Subtract the numerators: $(5 - 1 = 4)$
2. Keep the common denominator.
3. Reduce the fraction by dividing by the greatest common factor:

$$\frac{4}{6} \div \frac{2}{2} = \frac{2}{3}$$

Subtracting Fractions with Unlike Denominators

Example

$$\frac{5}{12} - \frac{1}{8} = ?$$

$$\frac{5 \times 2}{12 \times 2} = \frac{10}{24}$$

$$\frac{1 \times 3}{8 \times 3} = \frac{3}{24}$$

$$\frac{10}{24} - \frac{3}{24} = \frac{7}{24}$$

Steps

1. Find the LCD by listing the multiples of each denominator.
   - 12 {12, **24**, 36, 48}
   - 8 {8, 16, **24**, 32}
   - The LCD is 24.
2. Change the numerator to reflect the new denominator. (What is done to the bottom must be done to the top of a fraction.)
3. Subtract the new numerators: $10 - 3 = 7$. The denominator stays the same.

Borrowing from Whole Numbers

Example

$$4\frac{2}{3} - 3\frac{5}{7}$$

$$4\frac{2 \times 7}{3 \times 7} = 4\frac{14}{21}$$

$$\overset{3}{\cancel{4}}\frac{14}{21} + \frac{21}{21} = 3\frac{35}{21}$$

$$3\frac{5 \times 3}{7 \times 3} = 3\frac{15}{21}$$

$$3\frac{35}{21} - 3\frac{15}{21} = \frac{20}{21}$$

Steps

1. Find the LCD.
2. Fifteen cannot be subtracted from 14; therefore, 1 must be borrowed from the whole number, making it 3, and the borrowed 1 must be added to the fraction.
3. Add the original numerator to the borrowed numerator: $14 + 21 = 35$.
4. Now the whole number and the numerator can be subtracted.

SAMPLE PROBLEMS

Subtract the fractions in the following problems as indicated.

1. $\dfrac{5}{7} - \dfrac{2}{7} =$

2. $\dfrac{18}{24} - \dfrac{5}{24} =$

3. $\dfrac{2}{4} - \dfrac{3}{16} =$

4. $\dfrac{27}{56} - \dfrac{3}{7} =$

5. $1\dfrac{2}{5} - \dfrac{1}{2} =$

6. $16\dfrac{8}{9} - 5\dfrac{2}{3} =$

7. $11\dfrac{1}{5} - 8\dfrac{4}{5} =$

8. $20\dfrac{1}{2} - 4\dfrac{2}{3} =$

9. Terry has $8\frac{1}{4}$ feet of wood trim. He needs $5\frac{1}{3}$ feet of trim to decorate one wall. After cutting the wood to size, how much trim will Terry have left?

10. Jordan has a gallon of milk, which is equal to 16 cups. She uses $1\frac{1}{4}$ cups of milk to make pancakes. How much milk does Jordan have left after making pancakes?

Multiplication of Fractions

Example 1

$$\frac{2}{3} \times \frac{5}{8}$$

$$\frac{2}{3} \times \frac{5}{8} = \frac{10}{24} = \frac{5}{12}$$

Steps

1. Multiply the numerators together: $2 \times 5 = 10$.
2. Multiply the denominators together: $3 \times 8 = 24$.
3. Reduce the product by using the greatest common factor: $\dfrac{10 \div 2}{24 \div 2} = \dfrac{5}{12}$

Example 2

$$5 \times \frac{4}{13}$$

$$\frac{5}{1} \times \frac{4}{13} = \frac{20}{13} = 1\frac{7}{13}$$

Steps

1. Make the whole number 5 into a fraction by placing a 1 as the denominator.
2. Multiply the numerators: $5 \times 4 = 20$.
3. Multiply the denominators: $1 \times 13 = 13$.
4. Change the improper fraction into a mixed number.

Example 3

$$3\frac{1}{6} \times 6\frac{5}{8}$$

$$\frac{19}{6} \times \frac{53}{8} = \frac{1,007}{48}$$

$$\frac{1,007}{48} = 20\frac{47}{48}$$

Steps

1. Change the mixed numbers into improper fractions.

$$3\frac{+1}{\times 6} = (3 \times 6) + 1 = 19 \rightarrow \frac{19}{6}$$

$$6\frac{+5}{\times 8} = (6 \times 8) + 5 = 53 \rightarrow \frac{53}{8}$$

2. Multiply the numerators and denominators together.
   - $19 \times 53 = 1,007$ (numerator)
   - $6 \times 8 = 48$ (denominator)
   - Change the improper fraction into a mixed number.

$$48\overline{)1007} = 20\frac{47}{48}$$
$$\begin{array}{r} 20 \\ 48\overline{)1007} \\ -96 \\ \hline 47 \end{array}$$

Multiply the following fractions and reduce the product to the lowest form and/or mixed fraction (also referred to as the common denominator).

1. $\dfrac{3}{4} \times \dfrac{3}{6} =$

2. $\dfrac{2}{3} \times \dfrac{2}{8} =$

3. $5 \times \dfrac{7}{6} =$

4. $2\dfrac{6}{7} \times 7 =$

5. $5\dfrac{5}{8} \times 2\dfrac{5}{6} =$

6. $3\dfrac{1}{6} \times 1\dfrac{4}{5} =$

7. $2\dfrac{3}{4} \times 3 =$

8. $1\dfrac{3}{9} \times 3\dfrac{1}{4} =$

9. A baseball pitcher throws an average of 15 pitches per inning. This pitcher throws an average of 6⅓ innings per game. What is the average number of pitches per game for this pitcher?

10. Kelly's smart phone has a battery life of 10⅙ hours. She buys a new phone with a battery life that is 1½ times longer than her current phone. How many hours of battery life does her new phone have?

Division of Fractions

HESI Hint

"Dividing fractions, don't ask why, inverse the second fraction and then multiply."

Example:

$$\dfrac{1}{2} \div \dfrac{3}{8} \text{ Inverse } \dfrac{3}{8} \rightarrow \dfrac{8}{3}$$

$$\text{Then multiply } \dfrac{1}{2} \times \dfrac{8}{3}$$

$$\dfrac{1}{2} \times \dfrac{8}{3} = \dfrac{8}{6}$$

Write as an improper fraction: $1\dfrac{2}{6}$ then reduce to lowest form: $1\dfrac{1}{3}$

$$\dfrac{3}{8} \rightarrow \dfrac{8}{3} \quad \dfrac{3}{8} \times \dfrac{8}{3} = \dfrac{24}{24} = 1$$

These two numbers ($\dfrac{3}{8}$ and $\dfrac{8}{3}$) are **reciprocals** of each other because when they are multiplied together, they equal 1.

Example 1

$$\frac{1}{3} \div \frac{3}{4}$$

$$\frac{1}{3} \div \frac{3}{4}$$

$$\frac{1}{3} \times \frac{4}{3} = \frac{4}{9}$$

Steps

1. Inverse (or take the reciprocal) of the second fraction: $\frac{3}{4} \to \frac{4}{3}$.
2. Rewrite the new problem and multiply.
   - $1 \times 4 = 4$ (numerator)
   - $3 \times 3 = 9$ (denominator)

Example 2

$$1\frac{5}{6} \div \frac{3}{4}$$

$$1\frac{5}{6} \div \frac{3}{4}$$

$$\frac{11}{6} \div \frac{3}{4}$$

$$\frac{11}{6} \times \frac{4}{3} = \frac{44}{18}$$

$$2\frac{8}{18} = 2\frac{4}{9}$$

Steps

1. Change the mixed number into an improper fraction: $1\frac{5}{6} = (1 \times 6) + 5 = \frac{11}{6}$.
2. Rewrite the new problem with the improper fraction.
3. Inverse the second fraction.
4. Multiply the numerators and the denominators together.
   - $11 \times 4 = 44$ (numerators)
   - $6 \times 3 = 18$ (denominators)
5. Change the improper fraction into a mixed number. Reduce the mixed number.

Example 3

$$9 \div 3\frac{2}{3}$$

$$\frac{9}{1} \div \frac{11}{3}$$

$$\frac{9}{1} \times \frac{3}{11} = \frac{27}{11}$$

$$2\frac{5}{11}$$

Steps

1. Change the whole number into a fraction and the mixed number into an improper fraction.
2. Inverse the second fraction.
3. Multiply the numerators and then denominators together.
   - $9 \times 3 = 27$
   - $1 \times 11 = 11$
4. Change the improper fraction into a mixed number.

SAMPLE PROBLEMS

Divide the fractions in the following problems and reduce to the lowest common denominator.

1. $\dfrac{2}{3} \div \dfrac{1}{5} =$

2. $\dfrac{5}{12} \div \dfrac{2}{8} =$

3. $\dfrac{3}{8} \div \dfrac{2}{6} =$

4. $2 \div \dfrac{1}{7} =$

5. $6 \div \dfrac{2}{5} =$

6. $6\dfrac{2}{3} \div \dfrac{1}{3} =$

7. $7 \div 2\dfrac{1}{3} =$

8. $16\dfrac{2}{5} \div 4 =$

9. Gary has 1½ pounds of chicken. A recipe for chicken tacos allows for ⅛ pounds of chicken for each taco. How many tacos can Gary make?
10. Patty makes decorative wreaths. She has 31¼ feet of ribbon to make bows for her wreaths. Each bow requires 6¼ feet of ribbon. How many wreaths can Patty make?

Changing Fractions to Decimals

HESI Hint

"Top goes in the box, the bottom goes out."

   This is a helpful saying in remembering that the numerator is the dividend and the denominator is the divisor.

   If the decimal does not terminate, continue to the thousandths place and then round to the hundredths place.

   Example:

   7.8666 → 7.87

   If the number in the thousandths place is 5 or greater, round the number in the hundredths place to the next higher number. However, if the number in the thousandths place is less than 5, do not round up the number in the hundredths place.

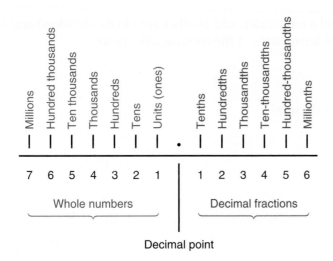

Millions | Hundred thousands | Ten thousands | Thousands | Hundreds | Tens | Units (ones) | . | Tenths | Hundredths | Thousandths | Ten-thousandths | Hundred-thousandths | Millionths

7 6 5 4 3 2 1   1 2 3 4 5 6

Whole numbers   Decimal fractions

Decimal point

Example 1

Change $\frac{1}{4}$ to a decimal.

$$\begin{array}{r} 0.25 \\ 4\overline{)1.00} \\ -8\downarrow \\ \hline 20 \\ -20 \\ \hline 0 \end{array}$$

Steps

1. Change the fraction into a division problem.
2. Add a decimal point after the 1 and add two zeros.
   - Remember to raise the decimal into the quotient area.
3. The answer is a **terminating decimal** (a decimal that is not continuous); therefore, adding additional zeros is not necessary.

Example 2

Change $\frac{5}{8}$ to a decimal.

$$\begin{array}{r} 0.625 \\ 8\overline{)5.000} \\ -48\downarrow\downarrow \\ \hline 20\downarrow \\ -16\downarrow \\ \hline 40 \\ -40 \\ \hline 0 \end{array}$$

Steps

1. Change the fraction into a division problem.
2. Add a decimal point after the 5 and add two zeros.
   - Remember to raise the decimal into the quotient area.

3. If there is still a remainder, add another zero to the dividend and bring it down.
4. The decimal terminates at the thousandths place.

Example 3

Change $\dfrac{1}{6}$ to a decimal.

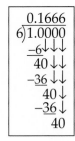

Steps

1. Change the fraction into a division problem.
2. After the 1, add a decimal point and two zeros.
3. The decimal continues (does not terminate); therefore, round to the hundredths place: $0.1666 \rightarrow 0.167$. (It can also be written as $0.1\overline{6}$. The line is placed over the number that repeats.)

Example 4

Change $3\dfrac{3}{4}$ to a decimal.

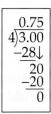

Steps

1. Change the fraction into a division problem.
2. After the 3, add a decimal and two zeros.
3. Place the whole number in front of the decimal: 3.75.

SAMPLE PROBLEMS

Change the following fractions into decimals and round to the nearest thousandth.

1. $\dfrac{1}{9}$

2. $\dfrac{1}{8}$

3. $\dfrac{5}{8}$

4. $\dfrac{2}{4}$

5. $\dfrac{2}{5}$

6. $1\dfrac{1}{4}$

7. $\dfrac{3}{12}$

8. $3\dfrac{3}{5}$

9. $9\dfrac{3}{16}$

10. $\dfrac{17}{25}$

Changing Decimals to Fractions

Example 1

Change 0.9 to a fraction.

$$0.9 \rightarrow \dfrac{9}{10}$$

Steps

Knowing place values makes it very simple to change decimals to fractions.
1. The last digit is located in the tenths place; therefore, the 9 becomes the numerator.
2. 10 becomes the denominator.

Example 2

Change 0.02 to a fraction.

$$0.02 \rightarrow \dfrac{2}{100} = \dfrac{1}{50}$$

Steps

1. The 2 is located in the hundredths place.
2. The numerator becomes 2, and 100 becomes the denominator.
3. Reduce the fraction.

Example 3

Change 0.75 to a fraction.

$$0.75 \rightarrow \dfrac{75}{100} = \dfrac{3}{4}$$

Steps

1. Always look at the last digit in the decimal. In this example, the 5 is located in the hundredths place.
2. The numerator becomes 75, and 100 becomes the denominator.
3. Reduce the fraction.

Example 4

Change 2.045 into a fraction.

$$2.045 \rightarrow 2\frac{45}{1000} \rightarrow 2\frac{9}{200}$$

Steps

1. The 5 is located in the thousandths place.
2. The numerator becomes 45, and 1,000 becomes the denominator. The 2 is still the whole number.
3. Reduce the fraction.

SAMPLE PROBLEMS

Change the following decimals into fractions and reduce to the lowest form.
1. $0.07 =$
2. $0.02 =$
3. $0.175 =$
4. $0.22 =$
5. $0.8 =$
6. $4.25 =$
7. $6.4 =$
8. $10.6667 =$
9. $8.24 =$
10. $0.075 =$

Ratios and Proportions

Ratio: A relationship between two numbers.
Proportion: Two ratios that have equal values.

HESI Hint

Ratios can be written several ways.
As a fraction: $\frac{5}{12}$
Using a colon: 5:12
In words: 5 to 12
Proportions can be written two ways.

$$\frac{5}{12} = \frac{25}{60}$$

$$5:12::25:60$$

NOTE: The numerator is listed first, then the denominator (known as the foil method).

Example 1

Change the decimal to a ratio.

$$.012 \rightarrow \frac{12}{1000} \rightarrow \frac{3}{250} \rightarrow 3:250$$

Steps

1. Change the decimal to a fraction.
2. Reduce the fraction.
3. The numerator (3) is the first listed number.
4. Then write the colon.
5. Finally, place the denominator (250) after the colon.

Example 2

Change the fraction to a ratio.

$$\frac{4}{5} = 4:5$$

Steps

1. The numerator (4) is the first listed number.
2. Then write the colon.
3. Finally, place the denominator (5) after the colon.

Example 3

Solve the proportion (find the value of x).

   $2:7 :: 8:x$

$$2:7 :: 8:x$$
$$\frac{2}{7} = \frac{8}{x}$$
$$\frac{2}{7} \overset{\times 4}{=} \frac{8}{x}$$
$$\frac{2}{7} = \frac{8}{x}$$
$$x = 28$$

Steps

1. Rewrite the proportion as a fraction (this might help to see the solution).
2. Note that $2 \times 4 = 8$; therefore, $7 \times 4 = 28$.
   - Multiply 7×8 (two diagonal numbers). The answer is 56.
   - $56 \div 2 = 28$ (Divide the remaining number.)
3. The answer is 28.

Example 4

Solve the proportion (find the value of x).

   $x:28 :: 12:48$

$$\frac{x}{28} = \frac{12}{48}$$
$$\frac{x}{28} = \frac{12}{48}$$
$$12 \times 28 = 336$$
$$336 \div 48 = 7$$
$$x = 7$$

Steps

1. Rewrite the proportion as a fraction.
2. Multiply the diagonal numbers: $12 \times 28 = 336$.

3. Divide the answer (336) by the remaining number: $336 \div 48 = 7$.
4. The value for x is 7.

Example 5

Solve the proportion (find the value of x).
     240:60 :: x:12.

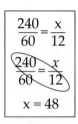

$$\frac{240}{60} = \frac{x}{12}$$

$$\frac{240}{60} = \frac{x}{12}$$

$$x = 48$$

HESI Hint

An example of the foil method is to remember "inside x inside and outside x outside."
     240:60 :: x:12
     60 times x :: 240 x 12
     60x :: 2,880
     Divide 60 by both sides to get x by itself
     x :: 48

Steps

1. Rewrite the proportion as a fraction.
2. Multiply the diagonal numbers together: $240 \times 12 = 2,880$.
3. Divide the answer (2,880) by the remaining number: $2,880 \div 60 = 48$.
4. The answer to x is 48.

SAMPLE PROBLEMS

Change the following fractions to ratios.

1. $\dfrac{12}{43}$

2. $\dfrac{7}{30}$

Solve the following for x:

3. $9:4 :: 117:x$
4. $3:11 :: x:99$
5. $x:12 :: 29:116$
6. $27:x :: 9:13$
7. $126:72 :: 14:x$
8. $x:144 :: 12:36$
9. If Barb types 130 words in 2 minutes, how long will it take her to type 325 words?
10. Steve is a painter. He needs 25 gallons of paint to cover 10 offices. Assuming all the offices are the same size, how many gallons of paint does Steve need to finish painting 3 offices?

Percentages

Percent: Per hundred (part per hundred).

Example 1

Change the decimal to a **percent:** 0.31 → 31%.

Steps

1. Move the decimal point to the right of the hundredths place (two places).
2. Put the percent sign behind the new number.

Example 2

Change the decimal to a percent: 0.007 → 0.7%.

Steps

1. Move the decimal point to the right of the hundredths place (always two places!).
2. Put the percent sign behind the new number. It is still a percent; it is just a very small percent.

Example 3

Change the percent to a decimal: 73.2% → 0.732.

Steps

1. Move the decimal two spaces away from the percent sign (to the left).
2. Drop the percent sign; it is no longer a percent, but a decimal.

Example 4

Change the percent to a decimal: 25% → 0.25.

Steps

1. The decimal point is not visible, but is always located after the last number.
2. Move the decimal two spaces away from the percent sign (toward the left).
3. Drop the percent sign; the number is no longer a percent, but a decimal.

Example 5

Change the fraction to a percent: $\dfrac{8}{9}$

$$
\begin{array}{r}
.888 \\
9\overline{)8.000} \\
-72\downarrow\downarrow \\
\hline
80\downarrow \\
-72\downarrow \\
\hline
80
\end{array}
$$

0.888 → 88.8%

Steps

1. Change the fraction into a division problem and solve.
2. Move the decimal behind the hundredths place in the quotient.
3. Place a percent sign after the new number.

Change the following decimals to percents.
1. 0.12 =
2. 0.04 =
3. 0.0052 =

Change the following percents to decimals.
4. 1.1% =
5. 8% =
6. 0.9% =

Change the following fractions to percents.
7. $\dfrac{7}{10}$ =

8. $\dfrac{2}{5}$ =

9. $\dfrac{5}{6}$ =

10. $\dfrac{1}{8}$ =

Using the Percent Formula

HESI Hint

The word *of* usually indicates the whole portion of the percent formula.
Percent formula:

$$\frac{\text{Part}}{\text{Whole}} = \frac{\%}{100}$$

Using this formula will help in all percent problems in which there is an unknown (solving for *x*).

Example 1

What is 7 out of 8 expressed as a percent?

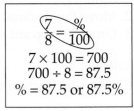

$$\frac{7}{8} = \frac{\%}{100}$$
$7 \times 100 = 700$
$700 \div 8 = 87.5$
$\% = 87.5$ or 87.5%

Steps

1. Rewrite the problem using the percent formula.
2. Multiply the diagonal numbers together: $7 \times 100 = 700$.
3. Divide by the remaining number: $700 \div 8 = 87.5\%$.

Example 2

What is 32% of 75?

$$\frac{x}{75} = \frac{32}{100}$$
$75 \times 32 = 2,400$
$2,400 \div 100 = 24$
$x = 24$

Steps

1. Rewrite the problem using the percent formula.
2. "Of 75:" 75 is the whole.
3. Multiply the diagonal numbers together: $75 \times 32 = 2{,}400$.
4. Divide by the remaining number: $2{,}400 \div 100 = 24$.
5. $x = 24$ (this is not a percent; it is the part).

Example 3

14 is 56% of what number?

$$\frac{14}{x} = \frac{56}{100}$$
$$14 \times 100 = 1{,}400$$
$$1{,}400 \div 56 = 25$$
$$x = 25$$

Steps

1. Rewrite the problem using the percent formula.
2. We are looking for the **whole** because *of* is indicating an unknown number.
3. Multiply the diagonal numbers together: $14 \times 100 = 1{,}400$.
4. Divide by the remaining number: $1{,}400 \div 56 = 25$.

Fractions, Decimals, and Percents

Fraction	Decimal	Percent
$\frac{1}{2}$	0.50	50%
$\frac{1}{4}$	0.25	25%
$\frac{3}{4}$	0.75	75%
$\frac{1}{5}$	0.20	20%
$\frac{2}{5}$	0.40	40%
$\frac{3}{5}$	0.60	60%
$\frac{4}{5}$	0.80	80%
$\frac{1}{8}$	0.125	12.5%
$\frac{3}{8}$	0.375	37.5%
$\frac{5}{8}$	0.625	62.5%
$\frac{7}{8}$	0.875	87.5%
$\frac{1}{3}$	0.333	33.3%
$\frac{2}{3}$	0.666	66.6%

SAMPLE PROBLEMS

Solve the following percent problems.
1. What is 14 out of 56 as a percent?
2. What is 2 out of 80 as a percent?
3. What is 45 out of 150 as a percent?
4. What is 50% of 90?
5. What is 85% of 40?
6. What is 2.5% of 400?
7. The number 5 is 20% of what number?
8. The number 30 is 25% of what number?
9. The number 9 is 30% of what number?
10. The number 51 is 25% of what number?

12-hour Clock versus Military Time

12-hour clock uses the numbers 1 through 12 with the suffixes am or pm to represent the hour in a 24-hour period. Military time uses the numbers 00 through 23 to represent the hour in a 24-hour period. The minutes and seconds in 12-hour clock and military time are expressed the same way.

HESI Hint

To convert to military time before noon, simply include a zero before the numbers 1 through 9 for AM. For example, 9:35 AM 12-hour clock time converts to 0935 military time. The zero is not needed when converting 10 AM or 11 AM. If the time is after noon, simply add 12 to the hour number. For example, 1:30 PM 12-hour clock time converts to 1330 military time (1 + 12 = 13). Midnight, or 12 AM, is converted to 0000. Noon, or 12 PM, is converted to 1200.

Table 1.1 summarizes the equivalents between military time and 12-hour clock time.

Military time is written with a colon between the minutes and seconds just as in the 12-hour clock. It can also be expressed with a colon between the hours and the minutes.

Table 1.1 Equivalents for Military Time and 12-hour Clock Time

Military Time	12-hour Clock Time	Military Time	12-hour Clock Time
0000	12:00 AM (Midnight)	1200	12:00 PM (Noon)
0100	1:00 AM	1300	1:00 PM
0200	2:00 AM	1400	2:00 PM
0300	3:00 AM	1500	3:00 PM
0400	4:00 AM	1600	4:00 PM
0500	5:00 AM	1700	5:00 PM
0600	6:00 AM	1800	6:00 PM
0700	7:00 AM	1900	7:00 PM
0800	8:00 AM	2000	8:00 PM
0900	9:00 AM	2100	9:00 PM
1000	10:00 AM	2200	10:00 PM
1100	11:00 AM	2300	11:00 PM

Military time is written as follows:

hours:minutes:seconds	OR	**hours:**minutes:seconds
0932:24 hours	OR	**09:**23:24
1926:56 hours	OR	**19:**26:56 hours

12-hour clock time is written as follows:
hours:minutes:seconds AM or PM
9:32:24 AM
7:26:56 PM

SAMPLE PROBLEMS

Convert the following 12-hour clock times to military times.
1. 12:01 AM =
2. 5:30 PM =
3. 6:10:17 AM =
4. 7:50:12 PM =
5. 2:23:15 PM =
6. 4:14:44 AM =

Convert the following military times to 12-hour clock times.
7. 1530 hours
8. 1908 hours
9. 11:10:22 hours
10. 02:08:33 hours
11. 1202:00 hours
12. 21:45:30

Algebra

Variable: A letter representing an unknown quantity (i.e., x).
Constant: A number that cannot change.
Expression: A mathematical sentence containing constants and variables (i.e., $3x - 2$).
Exponent: A number or symbol placed above and after another number or symbol (a superscript or subscript), indicating the number of times to multiply.

Algebra is a process that involves variables and constants. A **variable** is a letter that represents an unknown quantity. A **constant** is a number that cannot change. Using the operations of addition, subtraction, multiplication, and division, we can use algebra to determine the value of unknown quantities. Two algebra concepts discussed in this section will be evaluating **expressions** and solving equations for a specific variable.

HESI Hint

When working with algebra, remember to evaluate expressions by performing the "Order of Operations."

Order of Operations

1. Evaluate numbers within parentheses.	$4 \cdot (2 + 3)^2 - 5$
2. Multiply numbers based on any exponents.	$4 \cdot (5)^2 - 5$
3. Multiply and divide numbers from left to right.	$4 \cdot 25 - 5$
4. Add and subtract numbers from left to right.	$4 \cdot 25 - 5$

Continued

<u>**HESI Hint—cont'd**</u>

The variable for these expressions is 95.
Here's a mnemonic to remember the "Order of Operations":
    "Please excuse my dear Aunt Sally" helps to remember the correct order of operations.
    The order should be Parentheses, Exponents, Multiply, Divide, Add, Subtract.

Evaluating the Expression

- Numbers can be positive (1 or +1) or negative (–1). If a number has no sign (e.g., 1) it usually means it is a positive number.
- Adding positive numbers is similar to addition (e.g., $1 + 3 = 4$).
- Subtracting positive numbers is simple subtraction (e.g., $4 – 3 = 1$).
- Subtracting a negative number is the same as adding (e.g., $3 – [– 1] = 4$); it is written as $3 + 1 = 4$.
- Subtracting a positive number: $4 – (+3) = 4 – 3 = 1$
- Adding a negative number: $3 + (–4) = 3 – 4 = – 1$

Rules:

- Two like signs become positive signs: $3 + (+1) = 3(+1) = 3 + 1 = 4$

$$3-(-1)=3+1=4$$

- Two unlike signs become a negative sign: $8 + (– 2) = 8 – 2 = 6$

$$8-(+2)=8-2=6$$

When we substitute a specific value for each variable in the expression and then perform the operations, it's called "evaluating the expression."

Example 1

Evaluate the expression $ab + c$ if $a = 6, b = – 4$, and $c = 12$

$$(6)(-4)+12$$
$$-24+12$$
$$-12$$

Steps

1. Substitute the numbers into the given expression. Use parentheses when inserting numbers into an expression.
2. Multiply $6 \times -4 = -24$
3. Add $-24 + 12 = -12$

Example 2

Evaluate the expression $-xy(x-y)+y$ if $x=5$ and $y=-1$

$$-(5)(-1)([5]-[-1])+(-1)$$
$$-(-5)(5+1)-1$$
$$5(6)-1$$
$$30-1$$
$$29$$

Steps

1. Substitute the numbers into the given expression.
2. Multiply $5 \times -1 = -5$.
3. Change $-(-1)$ to $+1$, and $+(-1)$ to -1.
4. Add $5 + 1 = 6$
5. Change $-(-5) + 5$
6. Multiply $5 \times 6 = 30$
7. Subtract $30 - 1 = 29$

Solving Equations for a Specific Variable

To solve equations for a specific variable, perform the operations in the reverse order in which you evaluate expressions.

Example 3

Solve: $2x + 3 = 21$

$$\frac{\overset{-3}{2x}}{2} = \frac{\overset{-3}{18}}{2}$$

$$x = 9$$

Steps

1. Subtract 3 from each side of the equation.
2. Divide both sides by 2.

Example 4

Solve: $-4k - 2 = -17$

$$\frac{\overset{+2}{-4k}}{-4} = \frac{\overset{+2}{-15}}{4}$$

$$k = \frac{15}{4}$$

Steps

1. Add 2 to both sides.
2. Divide both sides by –4.
3. Simplify. (A negative divided by a negative is a positive.)

SAMPLE PROBLEMS

Evaluate the following expressions:
1. $x + 9y$ if $x = 3$ and $y = -2$
2. $2ab - am$ if $a = 1$, $b = 2$, and $m = -2$
3. $-2x(y - 2z)$ if $x = 3$, $y = -2$, and $z = 6$
4. $-qr + r - s$ if $q = 2$, $r = 4$, and $s = 6$
5. $(a + b)(2a + bc)$ if $a = 4$, $b = -2$, and $c = 3$
Solve the following equations for the given variable:
6. $6x - 6 = 24$ solve for x.
7. $-x - 4 = 18$ solve for x.
8. $4y + 15 = 28$ solve for y.

9. $2x + 18 = -4$ solve for x.

10. $-7 = 9a - 4$ solve for a.

Helpful Information to Memorize

Roman Numerals

I = 1	XX = 20	M = 1,000
II = 2	XXX = 30	V = 5,000
III = 3	XL = 40	X = 10,000
IV = 4	L = 50	L = 50,000
V = 5	LX = 60	C = 100,000
VI = 6	LXX = 70	D = 500,000
VII = 7	LXXX = 80	M = 1,000,000
VIII = 8	XC = 90	
IX = 9	C = 100	
X = 10	D = 500	
XI = 11		
Example 2012 = MMXII		

Measurement Conversions

Temperature
0° Celsius = 32° Fahrenheit (the freezing point of water)
Celsius to Fahrenheit
The temperature T in degrees Fahrenheit (°F) is equal to the temperature T in degrees Celsius (°C) times $\frac{9}{5}$ plus 32: $T_{(°F)} = T_{(°C)} \times 9/5 + 32$ or $T_{(°F)} = T_{(°C)} \times 1.8 + 32$ *Example* $T_{(°F)} = 20°C \times \frac{9}{5} + 32 = 68° F$
100° Celsius = 212° Fahrenheit (the boiling point of water)
Fahrenheit to Celsius
0 degrees Fahrenheit is equal to -17.77778 degrees Celsius: 0° F = -17.77778° C   The temperature T in degrees Celsius (°C) is equal to the temperature T in degrees Fahrenheit (° F) minus 32, times $\frac{5}{9}$: $T_{(°C)} = (T_{(°F)} - 32) \times \frac{5}{9}$ or $T_{(°C)} = (T_{(°F)} - 32) \div \left(\frac{9}{5}\right)$ or $T_{(°C)} = (T_{(°F)} - 32) \div 1.8$ **Example**   Convert 68 degrees Fahrenheit to degrees Celsius: $T_{(°C)} = (68°F - 32) \times \frac{5}{9} = 20° C$

Length	
Metric	*English*
1 kilometer = 1,000 meters	1 mile = 1,760 yards
1 meter = 100 centimeters	1 mile = 5,280 feet
1 centimeter = 10 millimeters	1 yard = 3 feet
2.54 centimeters = 1 inch	1 foot = 12 inches
Volume and Capacity	
Metric	*English*
1 liter = 1,000 milliliters	1 gallon = 4 quarts
1 milliliter = 1 cubic centimeter	1 gallon = 128 ounces
	1 quart = 2 pints
	1 pint = 2 cups
	1 cup = 8 ounces
	1 ounce = 30 milliliters (cubic centimeters)
Weight and Mass	
Metric	*English*
1 kilogram = 1,000 grams	1 ton = 2,000 pounds
1 gram = 1,000 milligrams	1 pound = 16 ounces
	2.2 pounds = 1 kilogram

ANSWERS TO SAMPLE PROBLEMS

Basic Addition and Subtraction

1. 1,471
2. 320
3. 2,001
4. 306
5. 232
6. 199
7. 398
8. 16,521
9. 7 blocks
10. 9

Basic Multiplication (Whole Numbers)

1. 984
2. 1,378
3. 18,062
4. 24,863
5. 71,550
6. 24,628
7. 65,067
8. 862,299
9. 1,656
10. 676

Basic Division (Whole Numbers)

1. 15
2. 2,100
3. 1,866
4. 21
5. 525
6. 975
7. 98.375
8. 1,256.2
9. 4.5
10. 15

Addition and Subtraction of Decimals

1. 11.14
2. 45.775
3. 210.2
4. 52.57
5. 19.26
6. 7.82
7. 57.91
8. 7.68
9. 15.25
10. 1.75

Multiplication of Decimals

1. 0.03924
2. 136.74
3. 24.644
4. 5,779.8
5. 7.408056
6. 148.4
7. 0.4068
8. 0.73572
9. 61.5 ounces
10. 4.8

Division of Decimals

1. 45
2. 180
3. 82
4. 62.2
5. 11.56
6. 4,560
7. 0.065
8. 2.4
9. 8
10. 4

Addition of Fractions

1. $\dfrac{7}{10}$

2. $\dfrac{5}{6}$

3. $1\dfrac{5}{6}$

4. $\dfrac{11}{16}$

5. $1\dfrac{32}{99}$

6. $11\dfrac{1}{12}$

7. $5\dfrac{32}{63}$

8. $8\dfrac{5}{18}$

9. $4\dfrac{1}{4}$

10. $148\dfrac{1}{6}$

Subtraction of Fractions

1. $\dfrac{3}{7}$

2. $\dfrac{13}{24}$

3. $\dfrac{5}{16}$

4. $\dfrac{3}{56}$

5. $\dfrac{9}{10}$

6. $11\dfrac{2}{9}$

7. $2\dfrac{2}{5}$

8. $15\dfrac{5}{6}$

9. $2\dfrac{11}{12}$ feet

10. $14\dfrac{3}{4}$ cups

Multiplication of Fractions

1. $\dfrac{3}{8}$

2. $\dfrac{1}{6}$

3. $5\dfrac{5}{6}$

4. 20

5. $15\dfrac{15}{16}$

6. $5\dfrac{7}{10}$

7. $8\dfrac{1}{4}$

8. $4\dfrac{1}{3}$

9. 95

10. $15\dfrac{1}{4}$

Division of Fractions

1. $3\dfrac{1}{3}$

2. $1\dfrac{2}{3}$

3. $1\dfrac{1}{8}$

4. 14

5. 15

6. 20

7. 3

8. $4\dfrac{1}{10}$

9. 12

10. 5

Changing Fractions to Decimals

1. 0.111
2. 0.125
3. 0.625
4. 0.5
5. 0.4
6. 1.25
7. 0.25

8. 3.6
9. 9.188
10. 0.68

Changing Decimals to Fractions

1. $\dfrac{7}{100}$

2. $\dfrac{1}{50}$

3. $\dfrac{7}{40}$

4. $\dfrac{11}{50}$

5. $\dfrac{4}{5}$

6. $4\dfrac{1}{4}$

7. $6\dfrac{2}{5}$

8. $10\dfrac{6667}{10000}$

9. $8\dfrac{6}{25}$

10. $\dfrac{3}{40}$

Ratios and Proportions

1. 12:43
2. 7:30
3. $x = 52$
4. $x = 27$
5. $x = 3$
6. $x = 39$
7. $x = 8$
8. $x = 48$
9. $x = 5$ minutes
10. $x = 7.5$

Percentages

1. 12%
2. 4%
3. 0.52%
4. 0.011
5. 0.08
6. 0.009

7. 70%
8. 40%
9. 83.333%
10. 12.5%

Using the Percent Formula

1. 25%
2. 2.5%
3. 30%
4. 45
5. 34
6. 10
7. 25
8. 120
9. 30
10. 204

12-hour Clock Time versus Military Time

1. 0001 hours OR 00:01 hours
2. 1730 hours OR 17:30 hours
3. 0610:17 hours OR 06:10:17 hours
4. 1950:12 hours OR 19:50:12 hours
5. 1423:15 hours OR 14:23:15 hours
6. 0414:44 hours OR 04:14:44 hours
7. 3:30 PM
8. 7:08 PM
9. 11:10:22 AM
10. 2:08:33 AM
11. 12:02:02 PM
12. 9:45:30 PM

Algebra

1. −15
2. 6
3. 84
4. −10
5. 4
6. $x = 5$
7. $x = -22$
8. $y = \dfrac{13}{4}$ or $y = 3\dfrac{1}{4}$ or $y = 3.25$
9. $x = -11$
10. $a = -\dfrac{1}{3}$

READING COMPREHENSION 2

Communication, whether written or spoken, sets us apart from all other life forms. We live in an age of instant telecommunication and think nothing of it. Yet, it is the written word that allows a person to record information that can travel across time and distance, to be examined and reexamined. In the health care setting, this is especially true for the health care provider as well as other members of the health care team as this is how information is shared among members of the health care team. The client record is written documentation of what is known of the client, including health care history, the evaluation or assessment, diagnosis, treatment, care, progress, and, possibly, the outcome. A clear understanding of all client information ensures better health care management for the client. The ability to skillfully read and understand also helps the health care personnel clearly document the client's written record as care is provided. Any student wishing to enter the health care profession must have the ability to read and understand the written word.

CHAPTER OUTLINE

KEY TERMS

Antonym
Assumption
Connotation
Context Clue

Inference
Purpose
Synonym
Tone

Identifying the Main Idea

Identifying the main idea is the key to understanding what has been read and what needs to be remembered. First, identify the topic of the passage or paragraph by asking the question, "What is it about?" Once that question has been answered, ask, "What point is the author making about the topic?" If the reader understands the author's message about the topic, the main idea has been identified.

In longer passages, the reader might find it helpful to count the number of paragraphs used to describe what is believed to be the main idea statement. If the majority of paragraphs include information about the main idea statement the reader has chosen, the reader is probably correct. However, if the answer chosen by the reader is mentioned in only one paragraph, the main idea that was chosen is probably just a detail.

Another helpful hint in identifying main ideas is to read a paragraph and then stop and summarize that paragraph. This type of active reading helps the reader focus on the content and can lessen the need to reread the entire passage several times.

Some students find that visualizing as they read helps them remember details and stay focused. They picture the information they are reading as if it were being projected on a bigscreen TV. If you do not already do this, try it. Informal classroom experiments have proved that students who visualize while reading comprehension tests easily outscore their counterparts who do not visualize.

HESI Hint

Main ideas can be found in the beginning, in the middle, or at the end of a paragraph or passage. Always check the introduction and conclusion for the main idea.

Finally, not all main ideas are stated. Identify unstated or implied main ideas by looking specifically at the details, examples, causes, and reasons given.

Again, asking the questions stated earlier will help in this task:
- What is the passage about? (Topic)
- What point is the author making about the topic? (Main idea)

Some experts like to compare the main idea with an umbrella covering all or most of the details in a paragraph or passage. The chosen main idea can be tested for accuracy by asking whether the other details will fit under the umbrella. The idea of an umbrella also helps visualize how broad a statement the main idea can be.

Identifying Supporting Details

Writing comprises main ideas and details. Few individuals would enjoy reading only a writer's main ideas. The details provide the interest, the visual picture, and the examples that sustain a reader's interest.

Often students confuse the author's main idea with the examples or reasons the author gives to support the main idea. These details give the reader a description, the background, or simply more information to support the writer's assertion or main idea. Without these details, the reader would neither be able to evaluate whether the writer has made his or her case nor would the reader find the passage as interesting. In addition to examples, facts and statistics may be used.

The reader's job is to distinguish between the details, which support the writer's main idea, and the main idea itself. Usually the reader can discover clues to help identify details because often an author uses transition words such as *one, next, another, first,* or *finally* to indicate that a detail is being provided.

Finding the Meaning of Words in Context

Even the most avid readers will come across words for which they do not know the meaning. Identifying the correct meanings of these words may be the key to identifying the author's main idea and to fully comprehending the author's meaning. The reader can, of course, stop and use a dictionary or a thesaurus for these words. However, this is usually neither the most efficient nor the most practical way to approach the unknown words.

There are other options the reader can use to find the meanings of unknown words, and these involve using context clues. The phrase **context clue** refers to the information provided by the author in the words or sentences surrounding the unknown word or words.

Some of the easiest context clues to recognize are as follows:

1. **Definition**—The author puts the meaning of the word in parentheses or states the definition in the following sentence.
2. **Synonym**—The author gives the reader another word that means the same or nearly the same as the unknown word.
3. **Antonym**—The author gives a word that means the opposite of the unknown word.

HESI Hint

The reader needs to watch for clue words such as *although, but,* and *instead,* which sometimes signal that an antonym is being used.

4. **Restatement**—The author restates the unknown word in a sentence using more familiar words.
5. **Examples**—The author gives examples that more clearly help the reader understand the meaning of the unknown word.
6. **Explanation**—The author gives more information about the unknown word, which better explains the meaning of the word.
7. **Word structure**—Sometimes simply knowing the meanings of basic prefixes, suffixes, and root words can help the reader make an educated guess about an unknown word.

HESI Hint

When being tested on finding the meaning of a word in the context of a passage, look carefully at the words and sentences surrounding the unknown word. The **context clues** are usually there for the reader to uncover. Once the correct meaning has been chosen, test that meaning in the passage. It should make sense, and the meaning should be supported by the other sentences in the passage or paragraph.

Identifying a Writer's Purpose and Tone

The purposes or reasons for reading or writing are similar for the readers and the writers. Readers read to be entertained, and authors write to entertain. Readers choose to read for information, and writers write to inform. However, in the area of persuasion, a reader can be fooled into believing he/she is reading something objective when in fact the author is trying to influence or manipulate the reader's thinking, which is why it is important for readers to ask the following questions:

1. Who is the intended audience?
2. Why is this being written?

If the writer is trying to change the reader's thinking, encourage the reader to buy something, or convince the reader to vote for someone, the reader can assume the writer's goal is to persuade. More evidence can be found to determine the writer's purpose by identifying specific words used within the passage. Words that are biased, or words that have positive or negative connotations, will often help the reader determine the author's reason for writing. (**Connotation** refers to the emotions or feelings that the reader attaches to words.)

If the writer uses a number of words with negative or positive connotations, the writer is usually trying to influence the reader's thinking about a person, place, or thing. Looking at the writer's choice of words also helps the reader determine the tone of the passage. (An author's **tone** refers to the attitude or feelings the author has about the topic.)

For example, if the author is writing about the Dallas City Council's decision to build waterways on the Trinity River bottom to resemble the San Antonio River Walk and describes this decision as being "inspired" and "visionary," the reader knows that the author has positive feelings about the decision. The tone of this article is positive because the words *inspired* and *visionary* are positive words. The reader might also be aware that the author may be trying to influence the reader's thinking.

On the other hand, if the writer describes the council's decision as being "wasteful" and "foolhardy," the reader knows the author has negative feelings about the council's decision. The reader can determine that the tone is unfavorable because of the words the writer chose. Typically, articles with obvious positive or negative tones and connotations will be found on the opinion or editorial page of the newspaper.

Articles or books written to inform should be less biased, and information should be presented in factual format and with sufficient supporting data to allow readers to form their own opinions on the event that occurred.

HESI Hint

When determining the writer's purpose and/or tone, look closely at the writer's choice of words. The words are the key clues.

Distinguishing between Fact and Opinion

A critical reader must be an active reader. A critical reader must question and evaluate the writer's underlying assumptions. An **assumption** is a set of beliefs that the writer has about the subject. A critical reader must determine whether the writer's statements are facts or opinions and whether the supporting evidence and details are relevant and valid. A critical reader is expected to determine whether the author's argument is credible and logical.

To distinguish between fact and opinion, the reader must understand the common definitions of those words. A fact is considered something that can be proved (either right or wrong). For example, at the time Columbus sailed for the New World, it was considered a scientific fact that the world was flat. Columbus proved the scientists wrong.

An opinion is a statement that cannot be proved. For example, "I thought the movie *Boyhood* was the best movie ever made" is a statement of opinion. It is subjective; it is the writer's personal opinion. On the other hand, the following is a statement of fact: "The movie *Boyhood* was nominated for an Academy Award for best picture in 2015 but did not win." This statement is a fact because it can be proved to be correct.

Again, the reader must look closely at the writer's choice of words in determining the fact or opinion. Word choices that include measurable data and colors are considered factual or concrete words. "Frank weighs 220 pounds" and "Mary's dress is red" are examples of concrete words being used in statements of fact.

If the writer uses evaluative or judgmental words *(good, better, best, worst)*, it is considered a statement of opinion. Abstract words *(love, hate, envy)* are also used in statements of opinion. These include ideas or concepts that cannot be measured. Statements that deal with probabilities or speculations about future events are also considered opinions.

Making Logical Inferences

In addition to determining fact and opinion, a critical reader is constantly required to make logical inferences. An **inference** is an educated guess or conclusion drawn by the reader based on the available facts and information. Although this may sound difficult and sometimes is, it is done frequently. A critical reader does not always know whether the inference is correct, but the inference is made based on the reader's own set of beliefs or assumptions.

Determining inferences is a skill often referred to as *reading between the lines.* It is a logical connection that is based on the situation, the facts provided, and the reader's knowledge and experience. The key to making logical inferences is to ensure that the inferences are supportable by evidence or facts presented in the reading. This often requires reading the passage twice so that details can be identified. Inferences are not stated in the reading but are derived from the information presented and influenced by the reader's knowledge and experience.

Summarizing

Identifying the best summary of a reading selection is a skill some students may find frustrating. Yet, this skill can be mastered easily when the following three rules are used:

1. The summary should include the main ideas from the beginning, middle, and end of the passage.
2. The summary is usually presented in sequence; however, occasionally it may be presented in a different order.
3. The summary must have accurate information. Sometimes a test summary will deliberately include false information. In that case, the critical reader will automatically throw out that test option.

Summary questions will typically take the longest for the student to answer because to answer them correctly, the student must go through each summary choice and locate the related information or main idea in the passage itself. Double-checking the summary choices is one way to verify that the reader has chosen the best summary. If the summary choice presents information that is inaccurate or out of order, the reader will automatically eliminate those choices.

HESI Hint

Remember, the summary should include the main ideas of the passage, possibly with some major supporting details. It is a shortened version of the passage that includes all the important information, eliminating the unnecessary and redundant.

REVIEW QUESTIONS

Recent advances in artificial intelligence (AI) have led to the development of Deep Learning (DL) systems. DL systems employ multilayered (deep) neural networks that function much like the human brain, allowing computers to grow and learn as they process vast amounts of data.

Medical applications of DL are currently generating intense interest. One area of study involves the role of DL technology in the identification of skin lesions. A research team at Stanford University developed a data base of nearly 130,000 images of skin lesions and fed the images, along with their diagnostic classifications, into a deep neural network. A study was then performed, pitting the machine against 25 dermatologists. The team concluded that the Stanford machine outperformed the dermatologists in correctly identifying skin lesions.

Such promising research in the field of medical AI has created understandable excitement. However, it is important to consider the potential risks and limitations of AI technology before its implementation is more fully realized. One concern involves overreliance on AI, which could result in a new breed of clinicians that lack essential diagnostic skills. Furthermore, concerns about privacy rights are likely to arise as more and more patient information is entered into these deep neural networks. Questions of liability must also be considered in the event that a diagnosis is missed by the computer.

But rather than resisting the implementation of medical AI, clinicians should seek opportunities to educate themselves and learn to work side by side with AI. One advantage for clinicians to consider is the benefit of increased efficiency. The Stanford machine was able to evaluate nearly 130,000 cases in about 3 months. Compare this with a dermatologist in full-time practice, who might see 200,000 cases during an entire lifetime. Additionally, dermatologists (and other clinicians) should consider the potential benefits of making clinical decisions with more confidence and greater accuracy with the help of AI.

1. What is the main idea of the passage?
   A. More research is needed before AI technology is used in clinical decision making.
   B. DL machines are better than dermatologists at identifying harmful skin lesions.
   C. Clinicians should consider the tremendous potential of DL systems and learn to work side by side with AI.
   D. Deep neural networks are capable of analyzing vast amounts of clinical data in a short amount of time.

2. Which fact is not listed as a detail in the passage?
   A. Stanford's machine evaluated nearly 130,000 cases in about 3 months.
   B. Stanford's machine outperformed 25 dermatologists in identifying skin lesions.
   C. AI technology has already resulted in lawsuits due to missed diagnoses.
   D. Deep neural networks are able to function much like the human brain.

3. In the third paragraph, the word *liability* refers to which area of concern?
   A. Legal responsibility
   B. Clinical accuracy
   C. Medical ethics
   D. Financial feasibility

4. What is the author's primary purpose in writing this essay?
   A. To encourage more research in the field of AI.
   B. To warn consumers about potential problems with DL machines.
   C. To educate clinicians about DL machines.
   D. To inform people about the potential benefits of AI in health care.

5. Identify the overall tone of the essay.
   A. Argumentative
   B. Optimistic
   C. Sympathetic
   D. Cautious

6. Which statement is an opinion?
   A. DL systems grow and learn as they process more data.
   B. Clinicians should learn to work side by side with AI machines.
   C. Medical applications of DL are generating intense interest.
   D. The Stanford machine was better at identifying skin lesions than dermatologists.

7. Which statement should be inferred by the reader?
   A. AI has the potential to change the way medical conditions are diagnosed.
   B. AI will soon take over "the dermatologist's" role in diagnosing skin lesions.

C. The risks of using AI in clinical diagnosis outweigh the benefits.

D. Clinicians will be worse at diagnosing diseases as a result of AI.

8. Choose the best summary of the passage.

A. AI technology has developed at a very rapid pace. Although initial research is promising, there are many issues that must be addressed before AI is put into wide use. Health care clinicians should be skeptical about the claims of AI researchers until more evidence is available.

B. The role of AI is expanding into the area of medical diagnosis. Research has shown that DL machines can increase the accuracy with which skin lesions are diagnosed. Health care clinicians should prepare themselves to take advantage of the potential benefits of AI technology.

C. The potential benefits of AI in the field of health care are virtually unlimited. Based on the latest research, DL machines are far better at diagnosing a disease than human clinicians. Cutting-edge AI technology should be implemented into daily clinical practice as quickly as possible.

D. As AI machines become smarter, they are able to process more and more data. The vast amount of patient information being fed into deep neural networks raises concerns about privacy rights. Clinicians should proceed with caution as they implement this new technology.

ANSWERS TO REVIEW QUESTIONS

1. C—main idea
2. C—supporting detail
3. A—meaning of word in context
4. D—author's purpose
5. B—author's tone
6. B—fact and opinion
7. A—inferences
8. B—summary

Bibliography

Johnson B: *The reading edge*, ed 4, New York, NY, 2001, Houghton Mifflin.

VOCABULARY

Members of the health professions use specific medical terminology to ensure accurate, concise, and consistent communication among all persons involved in the provision of health care. In addition to the use of specific medical terms, many general vocabulary words are used in a health care context. It is essential that students planning to enter the health care field have a basic understanding of these general vocabulary words to ensure accurate communication in a professional setting.

The following list of vocabulary words includes a definition for each word and an example of the word as used in a health care context. Careful study and review of these vocabulary words will help you begin your health profession studies with the ability to communicate in a professional manner.

Abstain: To voluntarily refrain from something.
Example: The dental hygienist instructed the patient to abstain from smoking to improve his breath odor.

Accountable: To be responsible.
Example: Paramedics are accountable for maintaining up-to-date knowledge of resuscitation techniques.

Acute: Sudden, intense.
Example: The nurse administered the prescribed pain medication to the patient who was experiencing acute pain after surgery.

Adhere: To hold fast or stick together.
Example: The tape must adhere to the patient's skin to hold the bandage in place.

Adverse: Undesired, possibly harmful.
Example: Vomiting is an adverse effect of many medications.

Ambivalent: Uncertain, having contradictory feelings.
Example: After learning that she had breast cancer, the patient was ambivalent about having a mastectomy.

Ambulate: To walk.
Example: The patient left the hospital as soon as he was able to ambulate independently.

Apply: To place, put on, or spread something.
Example: The nurse will apply a medication to the wound before covering the wound with a bandage.

Assent: To give consent; to agree.
Example: The patient was asked to assent to the surgery by signing the informed consent document.

Audible: Able to be heard.
Example: The respiratory therapist noted the patient's audible wheezing as a symptom of the patient's asthma.

Bacteria: Single-celled, microscopic organisms.
Example: The health care provider ordered a laboratory test to confirm that the patient's illness was caused by bacteria rather than a virus.

Bilateral: Present on two sides.
Example: The unlicensed assistive personnel reported to the nurse that the patient had bilateral weakness in the legs when walking.

Cardiac: Of or relating to the heart.
Example: Smoking increases the risk of cardiac disease.

Cavity: An opening or an empty area.
Example: The nurse inspected the patient's oral cavity for lesions.

Cease: Come to an end or bring to an end.
Example: Because the patient's breathing had ceased, the paramedic began resuscitation measures.

Chronic: Lasting or recurring over a long period of time.
Example: The patient has suffered from chronic headaches ever since a car accident 6 months ago.

Chronology: Order of events as they occurred; timeline.
Example: The police interviewed witnesses and first responders to determine the chronology of the accident.

Compensatory: Offsetting or making up for something.
Example: When the patient's blood pressure decreased, the paramedic noted that the heart rate increased, which was recognized as a compensatory action.

Concave: Rounded inward.
Example: The dietician noticed that the patient was very thin and that the patient's abdomen appeared concave.

Concise: Brief, to the point.
Example: When teaching a patient, the nurse tried to be concise so that the instructions would be easy to remember.

Congenital: Present at birth.
Example: The patient had surgery as a child to correct a congenital heart defect.

Consistency: Degree of viscosity; how thick or thin a fluid is in relation to how it flows.
Example: The respiratory therapist noticed that the mucus the patient was coughing was of a thin, watery consistency.

Constrict: To draw together or become smaller.
Example: The nurse knows that the small blood vessels of the skin will constrict when ice is applied to the skin.

Contingent: Dependent.
Example: The hygienist told the patient that a healthy mouth is contingent on careful daily brushing and flossing.

Contraindication: A reason something is not advisable or should not be done.
Example: The patient's excessive bleeding was a contraindication for discharge from the hospital.

Convulsive: Having or causing convulsions, i.e., violent shaking of the body.
Example: Epilepsy is a convulsive disorder.
Cursory: Quick, perfunctory, not thorough.
Example: During triage, the paramedic gave each accident victim a cursory examination.
Defecate: Expel feces.
Example: The unlicensed assistive personnel helped the patient to the toilet when the patient needed to defecate.
Deficit: A deficiency or lack of something.
Example: The therapist explained that the patient will experience a fluid deficit if the patient continues to perspire heavily during exercise without drinking enough fluids.
Depress: Press downward.
Example: The nurse will depress the patient's skin to see if any swelling is present.
Depth: Downward measurement from a surface.
Example: The nurse measures the depth of a wound by inserting a cotton swab into the wound.
Deteriorating: Worsening.
Example: The dental hygienist explains that the condition of the patient's gums is deteriorating and treatment by the dentist is needed right away.
Diagnosis: Identification of an injury or disease.
Example: The patient received a diagnosis of pancreatitis.
Diffuse: Spread over a large area; generalized.
Example: The patient's swelling was originally limited to a small area but is now diffuse.
Dilate: To enlarge or expand.
Example: When shining a light in the patient's eyes, the nurse looks to see if both pupils dilate in response to the light.
Dilute: To make a liquid less concentrated.
Example: The pharmacy technician suggests that the patient use fruit juice to dilute a bitter-tasting drug so that the medication will be easier to swallow.
Discrete: Distinct, separate.
Example: The paramedic observed several discrete bruise marks on the patient's body.
Distal: Distant; away from the center (such as of the body).
Example: The paramedic suspected that the patient had a dislocated knee and knew it was important to check a distal pulse in the ankle.
Distended: Enlarged or expanded from pressure.

Example: When a blood vessel is distended, the laboratory technician can easily insert a needle to obtain a blood sample.
Dysfunction: Impaired or abnormal functioning.
Example: Family dysfunction may increase when a member experiences an acute physical illness.
Empathy: Ability to share what others are feeling; understanding the feelings of another.
Example: After being diagnosed with cancer, the health care provider felt more empathy toward patients with cancer.
Equilibrium: Balance.
Example: The nurse suspected that an ear infection was the cause of the patient's lack of equilibrium.
Etiology: The origin or cause of a disease or condition.
Example: The nurse interviewed the patient to determine the etiology of the patient's food poisoning.
Exacerbate: To make worse or more severe.
Example: The physical therapist recognized that too much exercise would exacerbate the patient's breathing difficulties.
Exposure: To come in contact.
Example: The nurse taught the parents of a newborn to avoid exposure to people with severe infections.
Extension: Lengthening; unbending a joint.
Example: The physical therapist helped the patient perform extension and flexion exercises.
Fatal: Resulting in death.
Example: The emergency medical technicians arrived too late to save any lives at the scene of a fatal car accident.
Fatigue: Extreme tiredness, exhaustion.
Example: The dietician explained to the patient that eating more iron-rich foods may help reduce feelings of fatigue.
Febrile: Related to or caused by a fever.
Example: An elevated body temperature is a sign of a febrile infection.
Flexion: Bending a joint.
Example: Arthritis can make flexion of the fingers difficult.
Flushed: Reddened or ruddy appearance.
Example: The therapist observed that the patient's face was flushed after the patient completed the exercises.
Gastrointestinal: Of or relating to the stomach and the intestines.

Example: The patient was diagnosed with a gastrointestinal disease.

Hematologic: Of or relating to blood.

Example: Pregnancy can put a woman at risk for anemia, which is a hematologic disorder.

Hydration: Maintenance of body fluid balance.

Example: The medical assistant explains that adequate hydration helps keep skin soft and supple.

Hygiene: Measures contributing to cleanliness and good health.

Example: The dental assistant teaches patients about good hygiene practices to maintain strong teeth.

Impaired: Diminished or lacking some usual quality or level.

Example: The paramedic stated that the patient's impaired speech was obvious in the way she slurred her words.

Impending: Occurring in the near future, about to happen.

Example: The nurse manager increased the emergency room staffing in anticipation of accidents being caused by the impending snowstorm.

Impervious: Impenetrable, not allowing anything to pass through.

Example: Standard precautions require the use of impervious gloves when bodily fluids are handled.

Imply: To suggest without explicitly stating.

Example: The look on the administrator's face implied that she was happy about the results of the inspection.

Incidence: Occurrence.

Example: In recent years there has been an increased incidence of infections that do not respond to antibiotics.

Infection: Contamination or invasion of body tissue by pathogenic organisms.

Example: The health care provider prescribed antibiotics for the patient with a bacterial infection.

Infer: To conclude or deduce.

Example: When the patient started crying while receiving an injection, the nurse inferred that the patient was in pain.

HESI Hint

The terms *imply* and *infer* are often confused and used interchangeably, but they do not have the same meaning. Remember: The sender of a message *implies*, and the receiver of the message *infers*.

Inflamed: Reddened, swollen, warm, and often tender.

Example: The nurse observed that the skin around the patient's wound was inflamed.

Ingest: To swallow for digestion.

Example: The paramedic may contact the poison control center when providing emergency care for a child who has ingested cleaning fluid.

Initiate: To begin or put into practice.

Example: The nurse decided to initiate safety measures to prevent injury because the patient was very weak.

Insidious: So gradual as to not become apparent for a long time.

Example: The health care provider explained that the cancer probably started years ago but had not been detected because its spread was insidious.

Intact: In place, unharmed.

Example: The nurse observed that the patient's bandage was intact.

Intubate: To insert a tube into something (usually a patient's airway).

Example: The patient was unable to breathe effectively, so the health care provider had to intubate immediately.

Invasive: Inserting or entering into a body part.

Example: The laboratory technician is careful when obtaining blood samples because this invasive procedure may cause problems such as infection or bruising.

Kinetic: Of or related to movement.

Example: Kinetic energy from the battery of the medical assistant's tablet caused the device to feel warm to the touch.

Labile: Changing rapidly and often.

Example: Because the child's temperature was labile, the nurse instructed the unlicensed assistive personnel to check the temperature frequently.

Laceration: Cut; tear.

Example: After the accident, the paramedic examined the patient's lacerations.

Latent: Present but not active or visible.

Example: The latent infection produced symptoms only when the patient's condition was weakened from another illness.

Lateral: On the side.

Example: The physical therapist recommended exercises to help increase the strength of the patient's lateral muscles.

Lethargic: Difficult to arouse.
Example: The unlicensed assistive personnel observed that on the morning after a patient received a sleeping pill, the patient was too lethargic to eat breakfast.

Manifestation: An indication or sign of a condition.
Example: The dietician looked for manifestations of poor nutrition, such as excessive weight loss and poor skin condition.

Musculoskeletal: Of or relating to muscle and skeleton.
Example: As a result of overtraining, the athlete suffered a musculoskeletal injury.

Neurologic: Of or relating to the nervous system.
Example: The nurse checked the neurologic status of the patient who was brought to the emergency room after a motorcycle accident.

Neurovascular: Of or relating to the nervous system and blood vessels.
Example: Strokes and aneurysms are neurovascular disorders.

Nutrient: Substance or ingredient that provides nourishment.
Example: The dietician explains that fruits and vegetables contain nutrients that reduce the risk of some cancers.

Occluded: Closed or obstructed.
Example: Because the patient's foot was cold and blue, the nurse reported that the patient's circulation to that foot was occluded.

Ongoing: Continuous.
Example: The nurse instructed the patient that the treatment would be ongoing throughout the patient's entire hospital stay.

Oral: Given through or affecting the mouth.
Example: The patient's instructions stated "no oral fluids for 24 hours following surgery."

Otic: Of the ear.
Example: The health care provider prescribed an otic medication to treat the patient's ear infection.

Parameter: A characteristic or constant factor, limit.
Example: The dietician explained that the number of calories needed for energy is one of the important parameters of a healthy diet.

Patent: Open.
Example: The nurse checked to see whether the intravenous needle was patent before giving the patient a medication.

Pathogenic: Causing or able to cause disease.
Example: Viruses and bacteria are pathogenic organisms.

Pathology: Processes, causes, and effects of a disease; abnormality.
Example: The health care provider called to request the pathology report for her patient.

Posterior: Located behind; in the back.
Example: The dentist examined the posterior surface of the tooth for a cavity.

Potent: Producing a strong effect.
Example: The potent medication immediately relieved the patient's pain.

Potential: Capable of occurring or likely to occur.
Example: Because the patient was very weak, the physical therapist felt the patient had a high potential for falling.

Precaution: Preventive measure.
Example: The laboratory technician wore gloves as a precaution against blood contamination.

Precipitous: Rapid, uncontrolled.
Example: The paramedic assisted the pregnant woman during a precipitous delivery in her home.

Predispose: To make more susceptible or more likely to occur.
Example: The dietician explains that high dietary fat intake predisposes some people to heart disease.

Preexisting: Already present.
Example: The nurse notified the health care provider that the patient has a preexisting condition that might lead to complications during the emergency surgery.

Primary: First or most significant.
Example: The patient's primary concern was when he could return to work after the operation.

Priority: Of great importance.
Example: The laboratory technician was gentle when inserting the needle because it is a high priority to ensure that the patient does not experience excessive pain and discomfort during the procedure.

Prognosis: The anticipated or expected course or outcome.
Example: The health care provider explained that, with treatment, the patient's prognosis was for a long and healthy life.

Rationale: The underlying reason.
Example: To ensure that the patient will follow the diet instructions, the medical assistant explains the rationale for the low-salt diet.

Recur: To occur again.

Example: To ensure that a tooth cavity does not recur, the dental hygienist instructs the patient to use toothpaste with fluoride regularly.

Renal: Of or relating to the kidneys.

Example: The nurse closely monitored the oral intake and urinary output of the patient with acute renal failure.

Residual: Remaining, continuing.

Example: Patients often have residual weakness after suffering a stroke.

Respiration: Inhalation and exhalation of air.

Example: Exercise increases the rate and depth of an individual's respirations.

Retain: To hold or keep.

Example: The nurse administered a medication to prevent the patient from retaining excess body fluid, which might cause swelling.

Status: Condition.

Example: The paramedic recognized that the patient's status was unstable, which necessitated immediate transport to the nearest medical center.

Subcutaneous: Under the skin.

Example: The nurse administered the medication by subcutaneous injection.

Sublingual: Under the tongue.

Example: The patient was prescribed a sublingual medication for chest pain.

Supplement: To take in addition to or to complete.

Example: The dietician instructed the patients to supplement their diets with calcium tablets to help build strong bones.

Suppress: To stop or subdue.

Example: When the child's temperature decreased, the nurse checked to see if any medications had been given that would have suppressed the fever.

Symmetric (symmetrical): Being equal or the same in size, shape, and relative position.

Example: The paramedic observed that the movement of both sides of the patient's chest was symmetrical after the accident.

Symptom: An indication of a problem.

Example: The nurse recognized that the patient's weakness was a symptom of bleeding after surgery.

Syndrome: Group of symptoms that, when occurring together, reflect a specific disease or disorder.

Example: After reviewing the patient's symptoms, which included pain and tingling in the hand and fingers, the health care provider made a diagnosis of carpal tunnel syndrome.

Therapeutic: Of or relating to the treatment of a disease or a disorder.

Example: Therapeutic diets may include calorie and salt restrictions.

Toxic: Causing harm, poisonous.

Example: The pediatric health care provider recommended that the parents of a toddler keep all toxic substances out of the toddler's reach.

Transdermal: Crossing through the skin.

Example: The health care provider prescribed a transdermal nicotine patch for a patient participating in the smoking cessation program.

Transmission: Transfer, such as of a disease, from one person to another.

Example: Nurses should wash their hands to prevent the transmission of infections.

Trauma: Injury, wound.

Example: The accident victim had severe facial trauma.

Triage: Process used to determine the priority of treatment for patients according to the severity of a patient's condition and the likelihood of benefit from the treatment.

Example: When the paramedics arrived at the scene of the accident, they had to triage the patients.

Ubiquitous: Being or seeming to be everywhere at once.

Example: The patient noticed the ubiquitous "no smoking" signs in the clinic.

Urinate: Excrete or expel urine.

Example: The patient was instructed to urinate into the container so the nurse could send the urine sample to the laboratory.

Vascular: Of or relating to blood vessels.

Example: The patient underwent vascular surgery for the repair of an abdominal aortic aneurysm.

Virulent: Extremely harmful and severe.

Example: The virulent infection required an aggressive treatment regimen.

Virus: Microscopic infectious agent capable of replicating only in living cells, usually causing infectious disease.

Example: A person with a cold who goes shopping can transmit the virus to others.

Vital: Essential.

Example: The paramedic knows that it is vital to learn what type of poison was taken when caring for a poisoning victim.

Volume: Amount of space occupied by a fluid.

Example: The nurse recorded the volume of cough syrup administered to the patient.

REVIEW QUESTIONS

1. Select the meaning of the underlined word in the sentence. Certain bacterial infections are known to cause <u>diffuse</u> redness and swelling of the skin.
   A. Severe
   B. Painful
   C. Generalized
   D. Sudden

2. Select the meaning of the underlined word in the sentence. The nurse began to <u>triage</u> the patients so that the most critical injuries could be treated first.
   A. Discharge
   B. Transfer
   C. Admit
   D. Prioritize

3. What word meaning "sleepy" best fits in the sentence? The patient appeared _____ because she had only recently awoken from the anesthesia.
   A. Lethargic
   B. Impervious
   C. Ambivalent
   D. Ubiquitous

4. What is the best definition of the word *occluded*?
   A. Blocked
   B. Injured
   C. Impaired
   D. Bloated

5. What word meaning "rapid, steep" best fits in the sentence? The health care provider prescribed fluids to correct the patient's _____ drop in blood pressure.
   A. Acute
   B. Precipitous
   C. Ongoing
   D. Deteriorating

6. What is the best definition of the word *symmetric*?
   A. Continuous
   B. Significant
   C. Equal
   D. Impenetrable

7. Select the meaning of the underlined word in the sentence. The health care provider ordered pathology tests to help determine the <u>etiology</u> of the patient's illness.
   A. Cause
   B. Duration
   C. Severity
   D. Outcome

8. Select the meaning of the underlined word in the sentence. The medication was given <u>subcutaneously</u>.
   A. Into a muscle
   B. Into a vein
   C. Under the tongue
   D. Under the skin

9. Select the meaning of the underlined word in the sentence. The nurse provided education about foods that might <u>exacerbate</u> the patient's symptoms.
   A. Improve
   B. Reduce
   C. Prolong
   D. Worsen

10. Select the meaning of the underlined word in the sentence. The rescuer should make sure the victim's airway is <u>patent</u> before giving rescue breaths.
    A. Safe
    B. Working
    C. Open
    D. Visible

ANSWERS TO REVIEW QUESTIONS

1. C—Generalized
2. D—Prioritize
3. A—Lethargic
4. A—Blocked
5. B—Precipitous

6. C—Equal
7. A—Cause
8. D—Under the skin
9. D—Worsen
10. C—Open

4 GRAMMAR

In the United States, the ability to speak and write the English language using proper grammar is a sign of an educated individual. When people are sick and need information or care from individuals in the health professions, they expect health care workers to be professional, well-educated individuals. It is therefore imperative that everyone in the health care professions understands and uses proper grammar.

Grammar varies a great deal from language to language. English as a second language (ESL) students have an added burden to becoming successful. For example, nursing research literature indicates that ESL nursing students are at greater risk for attrition and failure of the licensing examination. However, this burden can be overcome by learning proper grammar.

CHAPTER OUTLINE

KEY TERMS

Adjective
Adverb
Clause (independent clause, dependent clause)
Cliché
Compound Sentence
Conjunction
Direct Object
Euphemism
Indirect Object
Interjection

Misplaced Modifier
Noun (common noun, proper noun, abstract noun, collective noun)
Participial Phrase
Participle
Phrase
Predicate
Predicate Adjective
Predicate Nominative
Preposition

Pronoun (personal pronoun, possessive pronoun)
Run-On Sentence
Sentence (declarative, interrogative, imperative, exclamatory)
Sentence Fragment
Sexist Language
Subject
Textspeak
Verb

This chapter describes the parts of speech, important terms and their uses in grammar, commonly occurring grammatical errors, and suggestions for successful use of grammar.

Eight Parts of Speech

The eight parts of speech are nouns, pronouns, adjectives, verbs, adverbs, prepositions, conjunctions, and interjections.

Noun

A **noun** is a word or group of words that names a person, place, thing, or idea.

Common Noun A common noun is the general, not the particular, name of a person, place, or thing (e.g., *nurse, hospital, syringe*).

Proper Noun A proper noun is the official name of a person, place, or thing (e.g., *Fred, Paris, Washington University*). Proper nouns are capitalized.

Abstract Noun An abstract noun is the name of a quality or a general idea (e.g., *persistence, democracy*).

Collective Noun A collective noun is a noun that represents a group of persons, animals, or things (e.g., *family, flock, furniture*).

Pronoun

A **pronoun** is a word that takes the place of a noun, another pronoun, or a group of words acting as a noun. The word or group of words to which a pronoun refers is called the *antecedent*.

The *students* wanted *their* test papers graded and returned to *them* in a timely manner.

The word *students* is the antecedent of the pronouns *their* and *them*.

Personal Pronoun A personal pronoun refers to a specific person, place, thing, or idea by indicating the person speaking (first person), the person or people spoken to (second person), or any other person, place, thing, or idea being talked about (third person).

Personal pronouns also express number in that they are either singular or plural.

We (first person plural) were going to ask *you* (second person singular) to give *them* (third person plural) a ride to the office.

Possessive Pronoun A possessive pronoun is a form of personal pronoun that shows possession or ownership.

- That is *my* book.
- That book is *mine*.
- That is *his* book.
- That book is *his*.

A possessive pronoun does not contain an apostrophe.

Adjective

An **adjective** is a word, phrase, or clause that modifies a noun (the *biology* book) or pronoun (He is *nice.*). It answers the question *what kind* (a *hard* test), *which one* (an *English* test), *how many* (*three* tests), or *how much* (*many* tests). Verbs, pronouns, and nouns can act as adjectives. A type of verb form that functions as an adjective is a **participle**, which usually ends in *-ing* or *-ed*. Adjectives usually precede the noun or noun phrase that they modify (e.g., *the absent-minded professor*).

Examples

Verbs: The *scowling* professor, the *worried* student, the *broken* pencil

Pronouns: *My* book, *your* class, *that* book, *this* class

Nouns: The *professor's* class, the *biology* class

Verb

A **verb** is a word or phrase that is used to express an action or a state of being. A verb is the critical element of a sentence. Verbs express time through a property called the *tense*. The three primary tenses are:

- Present—Mary *works*
- Past—Mary *worked*
- Future—Mary *will work*

Some verbs are known as "linking verbs" because they link, or join, the subject of the sentence to a noun, pronoun, or predicate adjective. A linking verb does not show action.

- The most commonly used linking verbs are forms of the verb *to be: am, is, are, was, were, being, been* (e.g., That man *is* my professor.).
- Linking verbs are sometimes verbs that relate to the five senses: *look, sound, smell, feel,* and *taste* (e.g., That exam *looks* difficult.).
- Sometimes linking verbs reflect a state of being: *appear, seem, become, grow, turn, prove,* and *remain* (e.g., The professor *seems* tired.).

HESI Hint

The following are examples of proper and improper grammar related to verb usage.

- It is important that Vanessa *send* [**not** sends] her resumé immediately.
- I wish I *were* [**not** was] that smart.
- If I *were* [**not** was] you, I'd leave now.

Adverb

An **adverb** is a word, phrase, or clause that modifies a verb, an adjective, or another adverb.

Examples

Verb: The physician operates *quickly*.
Adjective: The nurse wears *very* colorful uniforms.
Another Adverb: The student scored *quite* badly on the test.

Preposition

A **preposition** is a word that shows the relationship of a noun or pronoun to some other word in the sentence. A compound preposition is a preposition that is made up of more than one word. A prepositional phrase is a group of words that begins with a preposition and ends with a

Box 4.1 Commonly Used Prepositions

aboard	in
about	including
above	inside
across	into
after	like
against	minus
along	near
amid	of
among	off
around	on
as	onto
at	opposite
barring	out
before	outside
behind	over
below	past
beneath	pending
beside	plus
between	prior to
beyond	throughout
but (except)	to
by	toward
concerning	under
considering	underneath
despite	unlike
down	until
during	up
except	upon
following	with
for	within
from	without

noun or a pronoun, which is called the *object* of the preposition. Box 4.1 lists commonly used prepositions.

Examples: Prepositional Phrases

Sam left the classroom *at noon*.
The students learned the basics *of grammar*.

Conjunction

A **conjunction** is a word that joins words, phrases, or clauses. Words that serve as *coordinating* conjunctions are *and, but, or, so, nor, for,* and *yet* (e.g., The nurse asked to work the early shift, *but* her request was denied.).

Correlative conjunctions work in pairs to join words or phrases (e.g., *Neither* the pharmacist *nor* her assistant could read the physician's handwriting.).

Sometimes, *subordinating* conjunctions join two clauses or thoughts (e.g., *While* the nurse was away on vacation, the hospital flooded.). *While the nurse was away on vacation* is dependent on the rest of the sentence to complete its meaning.

Interjection

An **interjection** is a word or phrase that expresses emotion or exclamation. It does not have any grammatical connection to the other words in the sentence (e.g., *Yikes*, that test was hard. *Whew*, that test was easy.).

Nine Important Terms to Understand

There are nine important terms to understand: Clause, direct object, indirect object, phrase, predicate, predicate adjective, predicate nominative, sentence, and subject.

Clause

A **clause** is a group of words that has a subject and a predicate.

Independent Clause An independent clause expresses a complete thought and can stand alone as a sentence (e.g., *The professor distributed the examinations* as soon as the students were seated.). *The professor distributed the examinations* expresses a complete thought and can stand alone as a sentence.

Dependent Clause A dependent clause begins with a subordinating conjunction (Box 4.2) and

Box 4.2 Commonly Used Subordinating Conjunctions
after
because
before
until
since
when

does not express a complete thought and therefore cannot stand alone as a sentence. *As soon as the students were seated* does not express a complete thought. It needs the independent clause to complete the meaning and form the sentence.

Direct Object

A **direct object** is the person or thing that is directly affected by the action of the verb. A direct object answers the question *what* or *whom* after a transitive verb.
The students watched the professor distribute the examinations.
The professor answers *whom* the students watched.

Indirect Object

An **indirect object** is the person or thing that is indirectly affected by the action of the verb. A sentence can have an indirect object only if it has a direct object. An indirect object answers the question *to whom, for whom, to what,* or *for what* after an action verb.

Indirect objects come between the verb and direct object.
The professor gave his class the test results.
His class is the indirect object. It comes between the verb (*gave*) and the direct object (*test results*), and it answers the question *to whom*.

Phrase

A **phrase** is a group of two or more words that acts as a single part of speech in a sentence. A phrase can be used as a noun, an adjective, or an adverb. A phrase lacks a subject and predicate.

Predicate

A **predicate** is the part of the sentence that tells what the subject does or what is done to the subject. It includes the verb and all the words that modify the verb.

Predicate Adjective

A **predicate adjective** follows a linking verb and helps to explain the subject.

My professors are *wonderful*.

Predicate Nominative

A **predicate nominative** is a noun or pronoun that follows a linking verb and helps to explain or rename the subject.

Professors are *teachers*.

Sentence

A **sentence** is a group of words that expresses a complete thought. Every sentence has a subject and a predicate. There are four types of sentences.

Declarative A declarative sentence makes a statement.
Example: I went to the store.

Interrogative An interrogative sentence asks a question.
Example: Did you go to the store?

Imperative An imperative sentence makes a command or request.
Example: Go to the store.

Exclamatory An exclamatory sentence makes an exclamation.
Example: You went to the store!

HESI Hint

Many imperative sentences do not seem to have subjects. An imperative sentence often has an implied subject. For example, when we say *Stop that now,* the subject of the sentence, *you,* is implied *(You stop that now).*

Subject

A **subject** is a word, phrase, or clause that names whom or what the sentence is about.

Ten Common Grammatical Mistakes

Subject-Verb Agreement

A subject must agree with its verb in number. A singular subject requires a singular verb. Likewise, a plural subject requires a plural verb.

Incorrect: The nurses (plural noun) *was* (singular verb) in a hurry to get there.

Correct: The nurses (plural noun) *were* (plural verb) in a hurry to get there.

There are times when the subject-verb agreement can be tricky to determine.

When the Subject and Verb Are Separated

Find the subject and verb and make sure they agree.

Incorrect: The *question* that appears on all of the tests *are* inappropriate.

Correct: The *question* that appears on all of the tests *is* inappropriate.

Ignore any intervening phrases or clauses. Ignore words such as *including, along with, as well as, together with, besides, except*, and *plus*.

Example: The *dean*, along with his classes, *is* going on the tour of the facility.

Example: The *deans*, along with their classes, *are* going on the tour.

When the Subject Is a Collective Noun

A collective noun is singular in form but plural in meaning. It is a noun that represents a group of persons, animals, or things (e.g., *family, audience, committee, board, faculty, herd, flock*).

If the group is acting as a single entity, use a singular verb.

Example: The *faculty agrees* to administer the test.

If the group is acting separately, use a plural verb.

Example: The *faculty are* not in agreement about which test to administer.

When the Subject Is a Compound Subject

Usually, when the subject consists of two or more words that are connected by the word *and*, the subject is plural and calls for a plural verb.

Example: The *faculty* and the *students are* in the auditorium.

When the subject consists of two or more singular words that are connected by the words *or, either/or, neither/nor*, or *not only/but also*, the subject is singular and calls for a singular verb.

Example: Neither the *student* nor the *dean was* on time for class.

When the subject consists of singular and plural words that are connected by the words *or, either/or, neither/nor,* or *not only/but also,* choose a verb that agrees with the subject that is closest to the verb.

Example: Either the students or the teaching assistant is responsible.

Comma in a Compound Sentence

A **compound sentence** is a sentence that has two or more independent clauses. Each independent clause has a subject and a predicate and can stand alone as a sentence. When two independent clauses are joined by a coordinating conjunction such as *and, but, or,* or *nor,* place a comma before the conjunction.

Example: The professor thought the test was too easy, *but* the students thought it was too hard.

Run-On Sentence

A **run-on sentence** occurs when two or more complete sentences are written as though they were one sentence.

Example: The professor thought the test was too easy the students thought it was too hard.

A comma splice is one kind of run-on sentence. It occurs when two independent clauses are joined by only a comma.

Example: The professor thought the test was too easy, the students thought it was too hard.

The problem can be solved by replacing the comma with a dash, a semicolon, or a colon; by adding a coordinating conjunction; or by making two separate sentences.

Pronoun Case

Is it correct to say, "It was *me*" or "It was *I*"; "It must be *they*" or "It must be *them*"?

The correct pronoun to use depends on the pronoun's case. *Case* refers to the form of a noun or pronoun that indicates its relation to the other words in a sentence. There are three cases: *nominative, objective,* and *possessive.* The case of a personal pronoun depends on the pronoun's function in the sentence. The pronoun can function as a subject, a complement (predicate nominative, direct object, or indirect object), an object

of a preposition, or a replacement for a possessive noun.

Examples: Pronoun Use

- When the pronoun is the subject
  I studied for the examination.
  I is the subject of the sentence. Therefore, use the nominative form of the pronoun.
- When pronouns are the subject in a compound subject
  Is it correct to say, **"He and I** went to the conference" or **"Him and me** went to the conference"?
  Is it accurate to say, **"John and me** worked through the night" or **"John and I** worked through the night"?
  Is it proper to say, **"Her and Maria** liked the chocolate-covered toffee" or **"She and Maria** liked the chocolate-covered toffee"?

Knowing which pronoun is accurate requires understanding of how the pronoun is used in the sentence, so we know to use the nominative case. Therefore *He and I, I,* and *She* are the accurate forms of the pronouns.

HESI Hint

When choosing a pronoun that is in a compound subject, sometimes it is helpful to say the sentence without the conjunction and the other subject. We would not say, *Him* went to the conference or *Me* worked through the night or *Her* liked the chocolate-covered toffee. We would, however, say, *He* went to the conference and *I* worked through the night and *She* liked the chocolate-covered toffee.

HESI Hint

It is considered polite to place the pronoun *I* last in a series: *Luke, Jo, and I strive to do a good job.*

- When the pronoun is the object of the preposition
  Susan gave the results of the test to them.
  The pronoun *them* is the object of the preposition *to.* When the object of the preposition is a compound object, as in *"Susan gave the results of the test to Jo and me,"* the objective form of the pronoun is used.
- When the pronoun replaces a possessive noun
  That desk is hers.
  The possessive pronoun *hers* is used to replace a possessive noun. For example, suppose there is a desk that belongs to Holly. We would say,

That desk belongs to Holly. That is Holly's desk. That desk is Holly's. That desk is hers.

Pronouns that Indicate Possession

The possessive forms of personal pronouns have their own possessive forms, as shown in Table 4.1. Do not confuse these possessive pronouns with contractions that are similarly pronounced or spelled. Examples are shown in Table 4.2.

Incorrect Apostrophe Usage

Apostrophes are used to show possession or to show that letters have been omitted (i.e., a contraction). Apostrophes are not used to make a word plural, including years and surnames.
Examples of plurals: during the 1980s, from the Smiths, with the Inezes
Examples of possessives:
    Singular: 1980's highest grossing film, Mr. Smith's home, Inez's car
    Plural: the 1980s' highest grossing film, the Smiths' home, the Inezes' cars

Comma in a Series

Use a comma to separate three or more items in a series or list. A famous dedication makes the problem apparent: "To my parents, Ayn Rand and God." Because of the comma placement, it appears as though Ayn Rand and God are the parents. Place a comma between each item in the list and before the conjunction to avoid confusion.
Example: The nursing student took classes in English, biology, and chemistry.

Unclear or Vague Pronoun Reference

An unclear or vague pronoun reference makes a sentence confusing and difficult to understand.
Example: The teacher and the student knew that she was wrong.
    Who was wrong: the teacher or the student? The meaning is unclear. Rewrite the sentence to avoid confusion.
Example: The teacher and the student knew that the *student* was wrong.

Sentence Fragments

Sentence fragments are incomplete sentences.
Example: While the students were taking the test.
    The students were taking the test is a complete sentence. However, use of the word *while* turns it into a dependent clause. In order to make the fragment a sentence, it is necessary to supply an independent clause.
Example: While the students were taking the test, the professor walked around the classroom.

Misplaced Modifier

Misplaced modifiers are words or groups of words that are not located properly in relation to the words they modify.
Example: I fear my teaching assistant may have discarded the test I was grading in the trash can.

Table 4.1 Possessive Personal Pronouns

Pronoun	Possessive Forms	
I	My	Mine
He	His	His
She	Her	Hers
We	Our	Ours
You	Your	Yours
They	Their	Theirs
It	Its	Its

Table 4.2 Common Possessive Pronouns and Similar Contractions

Possessive Pronoun	Contraction
Its (belonging to *it*)	It's (it is, it has)
Their (belonging to *them*)	They're (they are)
Whose (belonging to *whom*)	Who's (who is, who has)
Your (belonging to *you*)	You're (you are)

Was the test being graded in the trash can?

The modifier *in the trash can* has been misplaced. The sentence should be rewritten so that the modifier is next to the word, phrase, or clause that it modifies.

Example: I fear the test I was grading may have been discarded in the trash can by my teaching assistant.

One type of misplaced modifier is a dangling participial phrase. A **participial phrase** is a phrase that is formed by a participle, its object, and the object's modifiers; the phrase functions as an adjective. A participial phrase modifies the noun that either directly precedes or follows the phrase. When the participial phrase directly precedes or follows a noun that it does not modify, the phrase is called a *dangling participial phrase.*

Example: Taking the patient's symptoms into account, a diagnosis was made by the physician.

The participial phrase *taking the patient's symptoms into account* is intended to modify the noun *physician;* however, because the phrase is placed closest to *diagnosis,* it appears to be modifying *diagnosis* instead of *physician.* Therefore, the sentence as it is written states that the diagnosis took the patient's symptoms into account, which is impossible.

Example: Taking the patient's symptoms into account, the physician made a diagnosis.

Five Suggestions for Success

Eliminate Clichés

Clichés are expressions or ideas that have lost their originality or impact over time because of excessive use. Examples of clichés are *blind as a bat, dead as a doornail, flat as a pancake, raining cats and dogs, keep a stiff upper lip, let the cat out of the bag, sick as a dog, take the bull by the horns, under the weather, white as a sheet,* and *you can't judge a book by its cover.*

Clichés should be avoided whenever possible because they are old, tired, and overused. If tempted to use a cliché, endeavor to rephrase the idea.

Eliminate Euphemisms

A **euphemism** is a mild, indirect, or vague term that has been substituted for one that is considered harsh, blunt, or offensive. In many instances, euphemisms are used in a sympathetic manner to shield and protect. Some people refuse to refer to someone who has died as "dead." Instead, they may say that the person has *passed away* or *departed.* Euphemisms should be eliminated, and we should try to speak and write more accurately and honestly using our own words whenever appropriate.

It is also essential to use accurate and anatomically correct language when referring to the body, a body part, or a bodily function. To do otherwise is unprofessional and tactless.

Eliminate Sexist Language

Sexist language refers to spoken or written styles that unnecessarily identify gender. Such language can suggest a sexist attitude on the part of the speaker or writer. In order to avoid stereotypes, try to use gender-neutral titles that do not specify a particular gender. Remember that inclusive language seeks to incorporate everyone who may be associated with a profession or group of people (e.g., use *police officer* instead of *policeman*).

HESI Hint

Attempts to eliminate sexist language may create grammatical problems if the word *his* or *her* is replaced with the word *their.* For example, *The doctor helps their patients.* However, this is grammatically incorrect because *their* is a plural pronoun that is being used in place of a singular noun. If the gender of the doctor is known, it is appropriate to use *his* or *her. The doctor helped her patients.* If the gender is not known, it is better to reword the sentence to avoid incorrect grammar as well as sexist language.
- Doctors help their patients.
- The patients are helped by their doctor.

Eliminate Profanity and Insensitive Language

Insensitive and obscene language can be insulting and cruel. What we say does make a difference. The nursery rhyme we learned in our youth, "Sticks and stones may break my bones, but words will never hurt me," is simply not true. Ask anyone who has been on the receiving end of language that is patronizing or demeaning. Because language constantly changes, sometimes we can be offensive without even realizing that we have committed a blunder. In the age of an "anything goes" attitude for television, music lyrics, and the Internet, it is difficult to know exactly what constitutes offensive language.

We need to be sensitive to language that excludes or emphasizes a person or group of people with reference to race, sexual orientation, age, gender, religion, or disability. We would all do well to remember another adage from childhood: The Golden Rule. Its message is clear: Respect the dignity of every human being, and treat others as you would like to be treated.

Eliminate Textspeak

Textspeak is language that is often used in text messages, emails, and other forms of electronic communication; it consists of abbreviations, slang, emoticons, and acronyms. With the pervasiveness of social media and text messaging, the use of textspeak may be second nature. However, it is important to be aware of when it is creeping into all electronic communication. Although textspeak is acceptable in informal communication, it is inappropriate to use textspeak in formal communication, such as in academic and professional settings. Just as use of proper grammar is taken as a sign of intelligence, use of textspeak can be taken as a sign of laziness.

Fifteen Troublesome Word Pairs

Affect versus Effect

Affect is normally used as a verb that means "to influence or to change" (The chemotherapy *affected* [changed] my daily routine.). As a noun, *affect* is an emotional response or disposition (The troubled teenager with the flat *affect* [disposition] attempted suicide).

Effect may be used as a noun or a verb. As a noun, it means "result or outcome" (The chemotherapy had a strange *effect* [result] on me). As a verb, it means "to bring about or accomplish" (As a result of the chemotherapy, I was able to *effect* [bring about] a number of changes in my life).

Among versus Between

Use *among* to show a relationship involving more than two persons or things being considered as a group (The professor will distribute the textbooks *among* the students in his class).

Use *between* to show a relationship involving two persons or things (I sit *between* Holly and Jo in class), to compare one person or thing with an entire group (What is the difference between this book and other grammar books?), or to compare more than two things in a group if each is considered individually (I cannot decide *between* the chemistry class, the biology class, and the anatomy class).

Amount versus Number

Amount is used when referring to things in bulk (The nurse had a huge *amount* of paperwork).
Number is used when referring to individual, countable units (The nurse had a *number* of charts to complete).

Good versus Well

Good is an adjective. Use *good* before nouns (He did a *good* job) and after linking verbs (She smells *good*) to modify the subject. *Well* is usually an adverb. When modifying a verb, use the adverb *well* (She plays softball *well*). *Well* is used as an adjective only when describing someone's health (She is getting *well*).

HESI Hint

To say that you feel well implies that you are in good health. To say that you are good or that you feel good implies that you are in good spirits.

Bad versus Badly

Apply the same rule for *bad* and *badly* that applies to good and well. Use *bad* as an adjective before nouns (He is a bad teacher) and after linking verbs (That smells bad) to modify the subject. Use *badly* as an adverb to modify an action verb (The student behaved *badly* in class).

Bring versus Take

Bring conveys action toward the speaker—to carry from a distant place to a near place (Please *bring* your textbooks to class).
Take conveys action away from the speaker—to carry from a near place to a distant place (Please *take* your textbooks home).

Can versus May (Could versus Might)

Can and *could* imply ability or power (I *can* make an A in that class). *May* and *might* imply permission (You *may* leave early) or possibility (I *may* leave early).

Farther versus Further

Farther refers to a measurable distance (The walk to class is much *farther* than I expected). *Further* refers to a figurative distance and means "to a greater degree" or "to a greater extent" (I will have to study *further* to make better grades). *Further* also means "moreover" (*Further/Furthermore*, let me tell you something) and "in addition to" (The student had nothing *further* to say).

Fewer versus Less

Fewer refers to number—things that can be counted or numbered—and is used with plural nouns (The professor has *fewer* students in his morning class than in his afternoon class).
Less refers to degree or amount—things in bulk or in the abstract—and is used with singular nouns (*Fewer* patients mean *less* work for the staff). *Less* is also used when referring to numeric or statistical terms (It is *less* than 2 miles to school. He scored *less* than 90 on the test. She spent *less* than $400 for this class. I am *less* than 5 feet tall.).

Hear versus Here

Hear is a verb meaning "to recognize sound by means of the ear" (I *hear* the music playing). *Here* is most commonly used as an adverb meaning "at or in this place" (The test will be *here* tomorrow).

i.e. versus e.g.

The abbreviation *i.e.* (that is) is often confused with *e.g.* (for example); *i.e.* specifies or explains (I love to study chemistry, *i.e.*, the science dealing with the composition and properties of matter), and *e.g.* gives an example (I love to study chemistry, *e.g.*, chemical equations, atomic structure, and molar relationships).

Learn versus Teach

Learn means "to receive or acquire knowledge" (I am going to *learn* all that I can about nursing). *Teach* means "to give or impart knowledge" (I will *teach* you how to convert decimals to fractions).

Lie versus Lay

Lie means "to recline or rest." The principal parts of the verb are *lie, lay, lain,* and *lying.* Forms of *lie* are never followed by a direct object.

Examples
- I *lie* down to rest.
- I *lay* down yesterday to rest.
- I had *lain* down to rest.
- I was *lying* on the sofa.

Lay means "to put or place." The principal parts of the verb are *lay, laid, laid,* and *laying.* Forms of *lay* are followed by a direct object.

Examples
- I *lay* the book on the table.
- I *laid* the book on the table yesterday.
- I have *laid* the book on the table before.
- I am *laying* the book on the table now.

Which versus That

Which is used to introduce nonessential clauses, and *that* is used to introduce essential clauses. A nonessential clause adds information to the sentence but is not necessary to make the meaning of the sentence clear. Use commas to set off a nonessential clause. An essential clause adds information to the sentence that is needed to make the sentence clear. Do not use commas to set off an essential clause.

Example: The hospital, *which flooded last July,* is down the street.

In this case, the phrase *which flooded last July* is a nonessential clause that is simply providing more information about the hospital.

Example: The hospital *that flooded last July* is down the street; the other hospital is across town.

In this case, the phrase *that flooded last July* is an essential clause because the information distinguishes the two hospitals as the one that flooded and the one that did not.

Who versus Whom

Who and *whom* serve as interrogative pronouns and relative pronouns. An interrogative pronoun is one that is used to form questions, and a relative pronoun is one that relates groups of words to nouns or other pronouns.

Examples

- *Who* is getting an A in this class? (Interrogative)
- Susan is the one *who* is getting an A in this class. (Relative)
- To *whom* shall I give the textbook? (Interrogative)
- Susan, *whom* the professor favors, is very bright. (Relative)

Who and *whom* may be singular or plural.

Examples

- *Who* is getting an A in this class? (Singular)
- *Who* are the students getting As in this class? (Plural)
- *Whom* did you say is passing the class? (Singular)
- *Whom* did you say are passing the class? (Plural)

Who is the nominative case. Use it for subjects and predicate nominatives.

HESI Hint

Use *who* or *whoever* if *he, she, they, I,* or *we* can be substituted in the *who* clause.

Who passed the chemistry test? *He/she/they/I* passed the chemistry test.

Whom is the objective case. Use it for direct objects, indirect objects, and objects of the prepositions.

HESI Hint

Use *whom* or *whomever* if *him, her, them, me,* or *us* can be substituted as the object of the verb or as the object of the preposition in the *whom* clause.

To *whom* did the professor give the test? He gave the test to *him/her/them/me/us.*

Summary

Review this chapter and ask yourself whether your use of the English language reflects that of an educated individual. If so, congratulations! If not, study the content of this chapter, and your scores on the HESI Admission Assessment are likely to improve.

REVIEW QUESTIONS

1. Which of the following sentences is grammatically correct?
   - A. Before finishing the book, Karen knew how it would end.
   - B. Hiking up the mountain, my legs began to feel weary.
   - C. Speaking in public for the first time, sweat began to form on Ben's brow.
   - D. After being lost at sea for weeks, the coast guard located the missing boat.

2. Which word in the following sentence is an adverb? Although the line was long, Stephen patiently waited for his turn to ride the roller coaster.
   - A. Although
   - B. long
   - C. patiently
   - D. ride

3. Which word in the following sentence is an indirect object? David wasn't hungry, so he gave me his sandwich.
   A. David
   B. me
   C. his
   D. sandwich
4. Which sentence is grammatically correct?
   A. Please bring all the items which are on the list.
   B. You should avoid acidic foods which cause indigestion.
   C. I enjoy books about Rome and Venice, that are places I'd like to visit.
   D. Be sure to follow the instructions that your teacher gave you.
5. The following sentence contains which type of word or phrase?
   Please meet me ASAP.
   A. Textspeak
   B. Euphemism
   C. Possessive
   D. Plural
6. Select the best word for the blank in the following sentence. The organizer printed dozens of fliers and distributed them ___ the group of volunteers.
   A. along
   B. among
   C. between
   D. inside

7. Which word in the following sentence is a preposition? The musicians quickly tuned their instruments before the concert.
   A. The
   B. quickly
   C. their
   D. before
8. Which word in the following sentence should be replaced? A nurse should always perform hand hygiene before she makes contact with the patient.
   A. nurse
   B. perform
   C. she
   D. patient
9. Select the best word for the blank in the following sentence. If you don't take the medication as directed, it will not have the desired _____ on your health.
   A. affect
   B. effect
   C. effectiveness
   D. affectiveness
10. What word is used incorrectly in this sentence? Its too soon to tell whether Janice's baby is a boy or a girl.
   A. Its
   B. too
   C. whether
   D. Janice's

ANSWERS TO REVIEW QUESTIONS

1. A—In this sentence, *before finishing the book* is a participial phrase that modifies Karen. The other sentences contain misplaced modifiers.
2. C—*Patiently* is an adverb that modifies *waited*.
3. B—An indirect object is the person or thing indirectly affected by the action of the verb. Indirect objects come between the verb and the direct object. In this sentence, the indirect object *me* receives the direct object *sandwich*.
4. D—*That* is used to introduce essential clauses. *Which* is most often used to introduce nonessential clauses (nonessential clauses are set off by commas). In this sentence, *that your teacher gave you* is an essential clause.
5. A—ASAP (As Soon As Possible) is an example of textspeak.

6. B—In this sentence, *among* is the correct choice because the fliers are being distributed to a group of people.
7. D—In this sentence, *before* is used as a preposition of time.
8. C—The use of the pronoun *she* in the sentence is an example of sexist language. This problem can be avoided by making the subject plural (nurses) and employing a gender-neutral pronoun: *Nurses should always perform hand hygiene before they make contact with the patient.*
9. B—The correct word for this sentence is *effect*, which is a noun that means "a result of something." *Affect* is most often used as a verb that means "to influence or to change."
10. A— *Its* is a possessive pronoun. The correct word for the beginning of this sentence is the contraction *It's*, meaning "it is."

5 | BIOLOGY

Biology is the scientific study of life; therefore, comprehending its basic components is important for understanding injuries and diseases. Members of the health professions naturally deal with biology, whether it requires knowing the structure of a cell, understanding how a molecule will react to a medication or treatment, or comprehending how certain organisms in the body function. Prospective students desiring to enter one of the health professions should have a basic knowledge of biology.

This chapter reviews the structure and reactions of cells and molecules. The concepts of cellular respiration, photosynthesis, cellular reproduction, and genetics are also presented.

CHAPTER OUTLINE

Biology Basics
Water
Biologic Molecules
Metabolism

The Cell
   Cellular Respiration
   Photosynthesis
Cellular Reproduction

Genetics
DNA
Review Questions
Answers to Review Questions

KEY TERMS

Alleles
Amino Acids
Binary Fission
Chromosomes
Citric Acid Cycle (also called Krebs Cycle)
Codon
Cytokinesis
Deoxyribonucleic Acid (DNA)
Electron Transport Chain
Glycolysis

Golgi Apparatus
Heterozygous
Homozygous
Interphase
Meiosis
Messenger RNA (mRNA)
Metabolic Pathway
Metaphase Plate
Mitosis
Organelles
Phagocytosis

Phospholipids
Photosynthesis
Punnett Square
Ribonucleic Acid (RNA)
Rough ER
Smooth ER
Steroids
Stop Codon
Transcription
Transfer RNA (tRNA)

Biology Basics

In biology, there is a hierarchic organizational system for nomenclature. In this system, kingdom is the largest and most inclusive category, while species is the most restrictive category. The order is as follows:

- Kingdom
- Phylum
- Class
- Order
- Family
- Genus
- Species

Science is a process. For an experiment to be performed, the following steps (commonly called the Scientific Method) must be taken:

- The first step is observation. New observations are made and/or previous data are studied.
- The second step is hypothesis, which is a statement or explanation of certain events or happenings.
- The third step is the experiment, which is a repeatable procedure of gathering data to support or refute the hypothesis.
- The fourth step in the scientific process is the conclusion where the data and its significance are fully explained.

Water

All life, and therefore biology, occurs in a water-based (or aqueous) environment. The water molecule consists of two hydrogen atoms covalently bonded to one oxygen atom. The most significant aspect of water is the polarity of its bonds that allow for hydrogen bonding between molecules. This type of intermolecular bonding has several resulting benefits. The first of these is water's high specific heat.

The specific heat is the amount of heat necessary to raise the temperature of 1 gram of that molecule by 1° Celsius. Water has a relatively high specific heat value due to the extent of hydrogen bonding between water molecules, which allows water to resist shifts in temperature. One powerful benefit is the ability of oceans or large bodies of water to stabilize climates.

Hydrogen bonding also results in strong cohesive and adhesive properties. Cohesion is the ability of a molecule to stay bonded or attracted to another molecule of the same substance. A good example is how water tends to run together on a newly waxed car. Adhesion is the ability of water to bond to or attract other molecules or substances. When water is sprayed on a wall, some of it sticks to the wall. That is adhesion.

When water freezes, it forms a lattice crystal. This causes the molecules to spread apart, resulting in the phenomenon of ice floating in water. Water is unique in this regard since most solids do not float on the liquid form of their substance because the molecules pack tighter in the solid form.

The polarity of water also allows it to act as a versatile solvent. Water can be used to dissolve a number of different substances (Fig. 5.1).

Biologic Molecules

There are multitudes of molecules that are significant to biology. The most important molecules are carbohydrates, lipids, proteins, and nucleic acids.

Carbohydrates

Carbohydrates are generally long chains, or polymers, of sugars. They have many functions and serve many different purposes. The most important of these are storage, structure, and energy. Carbohydrates form the backbone of important molecules such as deoxyribonucleic acid (DNA) and ribonucleic acid (RNA).

Lipids

Lipids are better known as fats, but specifically they are fatty acids, phospholipids, and steroids.

- **Fatty Acids** Fatty acids vary greatly but simply are grouped into two categories: saturated and unsaturated. Saturated fats contain no double bonds in their hydrocarbon tail. Conversely, unsaturated fats have one or more double bonds. As a result, saturated fats are solid, whereas unsaturated fats are liquid at room temperature. Saturated fats are those the general public considers detrimental; cardiovascular problems are likely associated with diets containing high quantities of saturated fats.
- **Phospholipids** Phospholipids consist of two fatty acids of varying length bonded to a phosphate group. The phosphate group is charged and, therefore, polar and soluble in water, whereas the hydrocarbon tail of the fatty acids is nonpolar and nonsoluble in water. This quality is particularly important in the function of cellular membranes. The

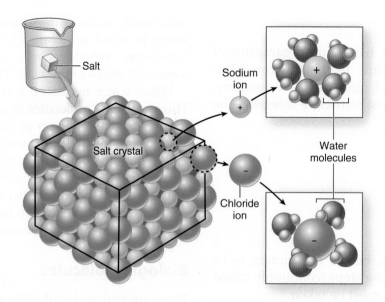

FIGURE 5.1 Water as a solvent. The polar nature of water (blue) favors ionization of substances in solution. Sodium (Na⁺) ions (pink) and chloride (Cl–) ions (green) dissociate in the solution. (From Patton KT, Thibodeau GA: *Anatomy and physiology*, ed 9, St Louis, 2016, Mosby.)

molecules organize in a way that creates a barrier that protects the cell.

- **Steroids** The last of the lipids are **steroids.** They are a component of membranes, but more important, many are precursors to significant hormones and drugs.

Proteins

Proteins are the most significant contributor to cellular function. They are polymers of 20 molecules called **amino acids.** Proteins are complex, consist of several structure types, and are the largest of the biologic molecules. Enzymes are particular types of proteins that act to catalyze different reactions or processes. Nearly all cellular function is catalyzed by some type of enzyme.

Nucleic Acids

Nucleic acids are components of the molecules of inheritance. **DNA** is a unique molecule specific to a particular organism and contains the code that is necessary for replication (Fig. 5.2). **RNA** is used in transfer of information from DNA to protein level and as a messenger in most species of the genetic code.

Metabolism

Metabolism is the sum of all chemical reactions that occur in an organism. In a cell, reactions take place in a series of steps called **metabolic pathways,** progressing from a standpoint of high energy to low energy. All of the reactions are catalyzed by the use of enzymes.

The Cell

The cell is the fundamental unit of biology. There are two types of cells: prokaryotic and eukaryotic cells. Cells consist of many components, most of which are referred to as **organelles.** Figure 5.3 illustrates a typical cell.

Prokaryotic cells lack a defined nucleus and do not contain membrane-bound organelles. Eukaryotic cells have a membrane-enclosed nucleus and a series of membrane-bound organelles that carry out the functions of the cell as directed by the genetic information contained in the nucleus. In other words, prokaryotic cells do not have membrane-bound organelles, whereas eukaryotic cells do. The eukaryotic cell is the more complex of the two cell types.

There are several different organelles functioning in a cell at a given time; only the major ones are considered here.

Nucleus

The first of the organelles is the nucleus, which contains the DNA of the cell in organized masses called **chromosomes.** Chromosomes contain all of the genetic information for the regeneration

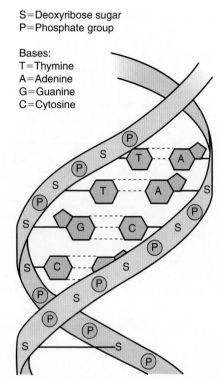

S=Deoxyribose sugar
P=Phosphate group

Bases:
T=Thymine
A=Adenine
G=Guanine
C=Cytosine

FIGURE 5.2 The DNA molecule. Representation of the DNA double helix showing the general structure of a nucleotide and the two kinds of "base pairs": adenine (A) with thymine (T) and guanine (G) with cytosine (C). (From Applegate: *The anatomy and physiology learning system*, ed 4, St Louis, 2011, Saunders.)

(repair and replication) of the cell, as well as all instructions for the function of the cell. Every organism has a characteristic number of chromosomes specific to the particular species.

Ribosomes

Ribosomes are organelles that read the RNA produced in the nucleus and translate the genetic instructions to produce proteins. Cells with a high rate of protein synthesis generally have a large number of ribosomes. Ribosomes can be found in two locations. Bound ribosomes are those found attached to the endoplasmic reticulum (ER), and free ribosomes are those found in the cytoplasm. The two types are interchangeable and have identical structures, although they have slightly different roles.

Endoplasmic Reticulum

The ER is a membranous organelle found attached to the nuclear membrane and consists of two continuous parts. Through an electron microscope, it is clear that part of the membranous system is covered with ribosomes. This section of the ER is referred to as **rough ER,** and it is responsible for protein synthesis and membrane production. The other section of the ER lacks ribosomes and is referred to as **smooth ER.** It functions in the detoxification and metabolism of multiple molecules.

Golgi Apparatus

Inside the cell is a packaging, processing, and shipping organelle that is called the **Golgi apparatus.** The Golgi apparatus transports proteins from the ER throughout the cell.

Lysosomes

Intracellular digestion takes place in lysosomes. Packed with hydrolytic enzymes, the lysosomes can hydrolyze proteins, fats, sugars, and nucleic acids. Lysosomes normally contain an acidic environment (around pH 4.5).

Vacuoles

Vacuoles are membrane-enclosed structures that have various functions, depending on cell type. Many cells, through a process called **phagocytosis,**

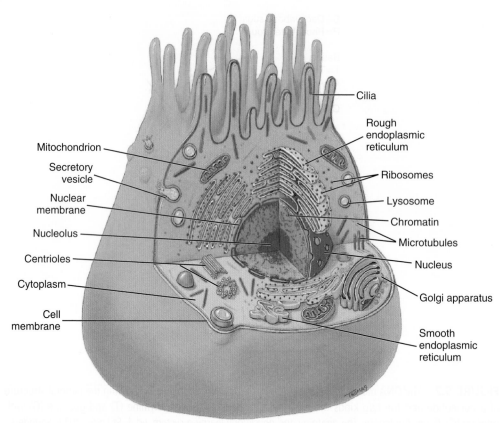

FIGURE 5.3 Generalized cell. (From Applegate: *The anatomy and physiology learning system,* ed 4, St Louis, 2011, Saunders.)

uptake food through the cell membrane, creating a food vacuole. Plant cells have a central vacuole that functions as storage, waste disposal, protection, and hydrolysis.

Mitochondria and Chloroplasts

There are two distinct organelles that produce cell energy: the mitochondrion and the chloroplast. Mitochondria are found in most eukaryotic cells and are the site of cellular respiration. Chloroplasts are found in plants and are the site of photosynthesis.

Cellular Membrane

The cellular membrane is the most important component of the cell, contributing to protection, communication, and the passage of substances into and out of the cell. The cell membrane itself consists of a bilayer of phospholipids with proteins, cholesterol, and glycoproteins peppered throughout. Because phospholipids are amphipathic molecules, this bilayer creates a hydrophobic region between the two layers of lipids, making it

selectively permeable. Many of the proteins, which pass completely through the membrane, act as transport highways for molecular movement into and out of the cell. Figure 5.4 illustrates the structure of the cellular membrane.

Cellular Energy Production

Cellular Respiration

There are two catabolic pathways that lead to cellular energy production. As a simple combustion reaction, cellular respiration produces far more energy than does its anaerobic counterpart, fermentation.

$$C_6H_{12}O_6 + 6O_2 \rightarrow 6CO_2 + 6H_2O$$

This balanced equation is the simplified chemistry behind respiration. The process itself actually occurs in a series of three complex steps that are simplified for our purposes.

There is one molecule that is used as the energy currency of the cell: adenosine triphosphate (ATP). Another compound that acts as a reducing agent and is a vehicle of stored energy is reduced

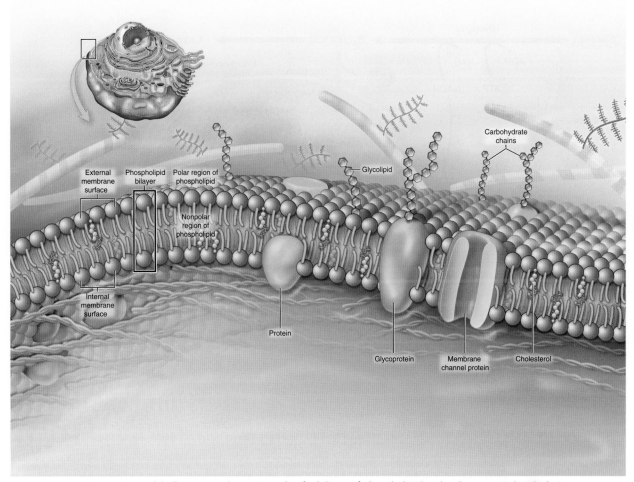

FIGURE 5.4 The plasma membrane is made of a bilayer of phospholipid molecules arranged with their nonpolar "tails" pointing toward each other. Cholesterol molecules help stabilize the flexible bilayer structure to prevent breakage. Protein molecules and protein-hybrid molecules may be found on the outer or inner surface of the bilayer—or extending all the way through the membrane. (From Patton KT, Thibodeau GA: *Anatomy and physiology*, ed 9, St Louis, 2016, Mosby.)

nicotinamide adenine dinucleotide (NADH). This molecule is used as a precursor to produce greater amounts of ATP in the final steps of respiration.

The first step in the metabolism of food to cellular energy is the conversion of glucose to pyruvate in a process called **glycolysis.** It takes place in the cytosol of the cell and produces two molecules of ATP, pyruvate, and NADH each.

In step two, the pyruvate is transported into a mitochondrion and used in the first of a series of reactions called the **citric acid cycle** (also called the Krebs cycle). This cycle takes place in the matrix of the mitochondria, and for a single consumed glucose molecule, two ATP molecules, six molecules of carbon dioxide, and six NADH molecules are produced.

The third step begins with the oxidation of the NADH molecules to produce oxygen and finally to produce water in a series of steps called the **electron transport chain.** The energy harvest here is remarkable. For every glucose molecule, 28 to 32 ATP molecules can be produced.

This conversion results in overall ATP production numbers of 32 to 36 ATP molecules for every glucose molecule consumed. For a summary of cellular respiration, see Figure 5.5.

Photosynthesis

In the previous section, the harvesting of energy by the cell was discussed. But where did that energy originate? It began with a glucose molecule

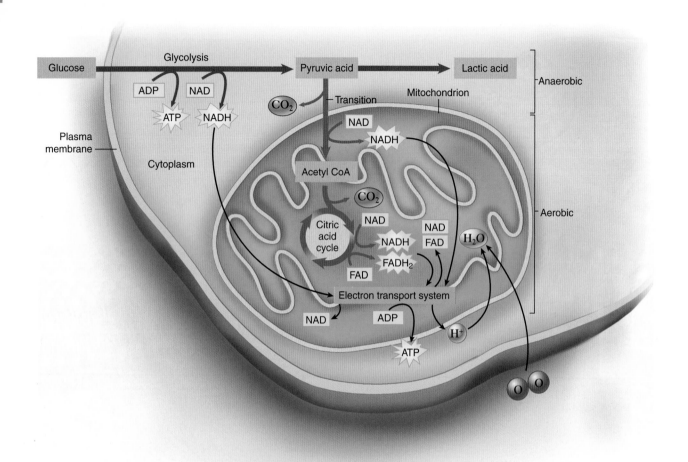

FIGURE 5.5 Summary of cellular respiration. This simplified outline of cellular respiration represents one of the most important catabolic pathways in the cell. Note that one phase (*glycolysis*) occurs in the cytosol but that the two remaining phases (*citric acid cycle* and *electron transport system*) occur within a mitochondrion. Note also the divergence of the anaerobic and aerobic pathways of cellular respiration. *ADP,* Adenosine diphosphate; *ATP,* adenosine triphosphate; *CoA,* coenzyme A; *FAD,* flavin adenine dinucleotide; *FADH$_2$,* form of flavin adenine dinucleotide; *NAD,* nicotinamide adenine dinucleotide; *NADH,* form of nicotinamide adenine dinucleotide. (From Patton KT, Thibodeau GA: *Anatomy and physiology,* ed 9, St Louis, 2016, Mosby.)

and resulted in a large production of energy in the form of ATP. A precursor to the glucose molecule is produced in a process called **photosynthesis.**

The chemical reaction representing this process is simply the reverse of cellular respiration.

$$6CO_2 + 6H_2O + \text{Light energy} \rightarrow C_6H_{12}O_6 + 6O_2$$

The only notable difference is the addition of light energy on the reactant side of the equation. Just as glucose is used to produce energy, so too must energy be used to produce glucose.

Photosynthesis is not as simple a process as it looks from the chemical equation. In fact, it

consists of two different stages: the light reactions and the Calvin cycle. The light reactions are those that convert solar energy to chemical energy. The cell accomplishes the production of ATP by absorbing light and using that energy to split a water molecule and transfer the electron, thus creating nicotinamide adenine dinucleotide phosphate and producing ATP. These molecules are then used in the Calvin cycle to produce sugar.

The sugar produced is polymerized and stored as a polymer of glucose. These sugars are consumed by organisms or by the plant itself to produce energy by cellular respiration.

When attempting to understand cell respiration and photosynthesis, keep in mind that these processes are cyclical. In other words, the raw materials for one process are the products of the other process. The raw materials for cellular respiration are glucose and oxygen, whereas the products of cell respiration are water, carbon dioxide, and ATP. Plants and other autotrophs will utilize the products of cell respiration (water, carbon dioxide) in the process of photosynthesis. The products of photosynthesis (oxygen, glucose) become the raw materials of cell respiration.

Cellular Reproduction

Cells reproduce by three different processes, all of which fall into two categories: sexual and asexual reproduction.

Asexual Reproduction

There are two types of asexual reproduction. The first involves bacterial cells and is referred to as **binary fission.** In this process, the chromosome binds to the plasma membrane where it replicates. Then as the cell grows, it pinches in two, producing two identical cells (Fig. 5.6).

Binary fission in bacteria

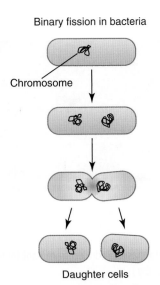

Chromosome

Daughter cells

FIGURE 5.6 Binary fission. A single cell separates into two identical daughter cells, each with an identical copy of parent DNA. (Redrawn from VanMeter K, et al: *Microbiology for the healthcare professional*, St Louis, 2010, Mosby.)

Another type of asexual reproduction is called **mitosis.** This process of cell division occurs in five stages before pinching in two in a process called **cytokinesis.** The five stages are prophase, prometaphase, metaphase, anaphase, and telophase.

During prophase, the chromosomes are visibly separate, and each duplicated chromosome has two noticeable sister chromatids. In prometaphase, the nuclear envelope begins to disappear, and the chromosomes begin to attach to the spindle that is forming along the axis of the cell. Metaphase follows, with all the chromosomes aligning along what is called the **metaphase plate** or the center of the cell. Anaphase begins when chromosomes start to separate. In this phase, the chromatids are considered separate chromosomes. The final phase is telophase. Here, chromosomes gather on either side of the now separating cell. This is the end of mitosis.

The second process associated with cell division is cytokinesis. During this phase, which is separate from the phases of mitosis, the cell pinches in two, forming two separate identical cells. A summary of mitosis is illustrated in Figure 5.7.

Sexual Reproduction

Sexual reproduction is different from asexual reproduction. In asexual reproduction, the offspring originates from a single cell, yielding all cells produced to be identical. In sexual reproduction, two cells contribute genetic material, resulting in significantly greater variation. These two cells find and fertilize each other randomly, making it virtually impossible for cells to be alike.

The process that determines how reproductive cells divide in a sexually reproducing organism is called **meiosis.** Meiosis consists of two distinct stages, meiosis I and meiosis II, resulting in four daughter cells (Fig. 5.8). Each of these daughter cells contains half as many chromosomes as the parent. Preceding these events is a period called **interphase.** It is during interphase that the chromosomes are duplicated and the cell prepares for division.

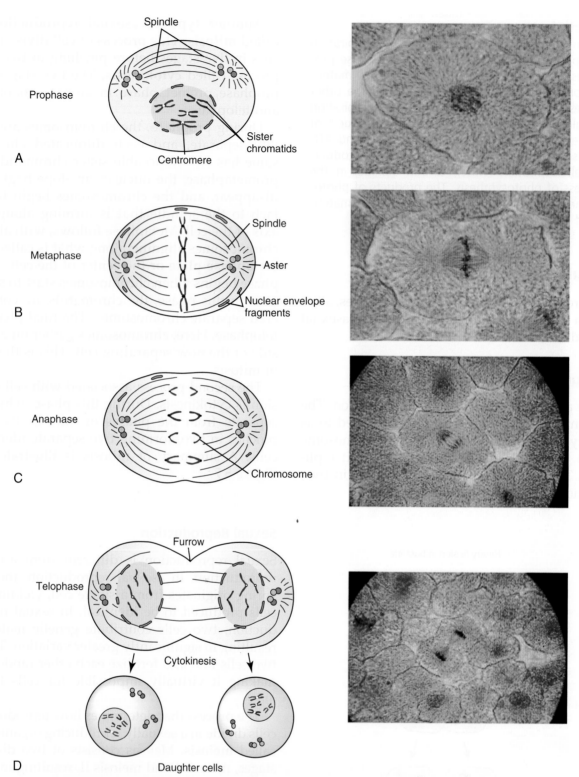

FIGURE 5.7 Mitosis. **A,** Prophase. **B,** Metaphase. **C,** Anaphase. **D,** Telophase. (Redrawn from VanMeter K, et al: *Microbiology for the healthcare professional,* St Louis, 2010, Mosby.)

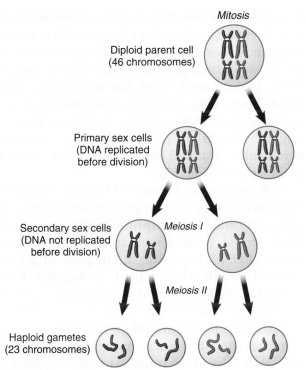

Mitosis

Diploid parent cell
(46 chromosomes)

Primary sex cells
(DNA replicated
before division)

Secondary sex cells
(DNA not replicated
before division)

Meiosis I

Meiosis II

Haploid gametes
(23 chromosomes)

FIGURE 5.8 Meiosis. Meiotic cell division takes place in two steps: *meiosis I* and *meiosis II*. Meiosis is called *reduction division* because the number of chromosomes is reduced by half (from the diploid number to the haploid number). (From Patton KT, Thibodeau GA: *Anatomy and physiology*, ed 9, St Louis, 2016, Mosby.)

Genetics

Using garden peas, Gregor Mendel discovered the basic principles of genetics. By careful experimentation, he was able to determine that the observable traits in peas were passed from one generation to the next.

From Mendel's studies, scientists have found that for every trait expressed in a sexually reproducing organism, there are at least two alternative versions of a gene called **alleles.** For simple traits, the versions can be one of two types: dominant or recessive. If both of the alleles are the same type, the organism is said to be **homozygous** for that trait. If they are different types, the organism is said to be **heterozygous.**

By using a device called a **Punnett square,** it is possible to predict genotype (the combination of alleles) and phenotype (what traits will be expressed) of the offspring of sexual reproduction. Alleles are placed one per column for one gene and one per row for the other gene. In the example in Figure 5.9, a homozygous dominant is crossed with a heterozygous organism for the same trait.

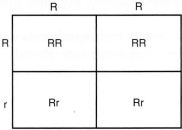

	R	R
R	RR	RR
r	Rr	Rr

FIGURE 5.9 Punnett square depicting the cross between a homozygous dominant and a heterozygous organism.

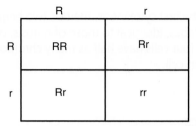

FIGURE 5.10 Punnett square depicting three possible dominant combinations.

Note that all progeny will express dominance for this trait. In the example in Figure 5.10, three of the possible combinations will be dominant, and one will be recessive for this trait.

The Punnett square can be used to cross any number of different traits simultaneously. With these data, a probability of phenotypes that will be produced can be determined. However, the more traits desired, the more complex the cross.

Not all genes express themselves according to these simple rules, but they are the basis for all genetic understanding. There are many other methods of genetic expression. A few of these include multiple alleles, pleiotropy, epistasis, and polygenic inheritance.

Because genetics is the study of heredity, many human disorders can be detected by studying a person's chromosomes or by creating a pedigree. A pedigree is a family tree that traces the occurrence of a certain trait through several generations. A pedigree is useful in understanding the genetic past as well as the possible future.

DNA

DNA is the genetic material of a cell and is the vehicle of inheritance. In 1953, Watson and Crick described the structure of DNA. They described a double helical structure that contains the four nitrogenous bases adenine, thymine, guanine, and cytosine.

Each base forms hydrogen bonds with another base on the complementary strand. The bases have a specific bonding pattern. Adenine bonds with thymine, and guanine bonds with cytosine. Because of this method of bonding, the strands can be replicated, producing identical strands of DNA. During replication, the strands are separated. Then, with the help of several enzymes, new complementary strands to each of the two original strands are created. This produces two new double-stranded segments of DNA identical to the original (Fig. 5.11).

Each gene along a strand of DNA is a template for protein synthesis. This production begins with a process called **transcription.** In this process, an RNA strand, complementary to the original strand of DNA, is produced. The piece of genetic material produced is called **messenger RNA (mRNA).** The RNA strand has nitrogenous bases identical to those in DNA with the exception of uracil, which is substituted for thymine.

mRNA functions as a messenger from the original DNA helix in the nucleus to the ribosomes in the cytosol or on the rough ER. Here, the ribosome acts as the site of translation. The mRNA slides through the ribosome. Every group of three bases along the stretch of RNA is called a **codon,** and each of these codes for a specific amino acid. The anticodon is located on a unit called **transfer RNA (tRNA),** which carries a specific amino acid. It binds to the ribosome when its codon is sliding through the ribosome. Remember that a protein is a polymer of amino acids, and multiple tRNA molecules bind in order and are released by the ribosome. Each amino acid is bonded together and released by the preceding tRNA molecule, creating an elongated chain of amino acids. Eventually the chain is ended at what is called a **stop codon.** At this point, the chain is released into the cytoplasm and the protein folds onto itself and forms its complete conformation.

By dictating what is produced in translation through transcription, the DNA in the nucleus has control over everything taking place in the cell. The proteins that are produced will perform all the different cellular functions required for the cell's survival. The synthesis of proteins is summarized in Figure 5.12.

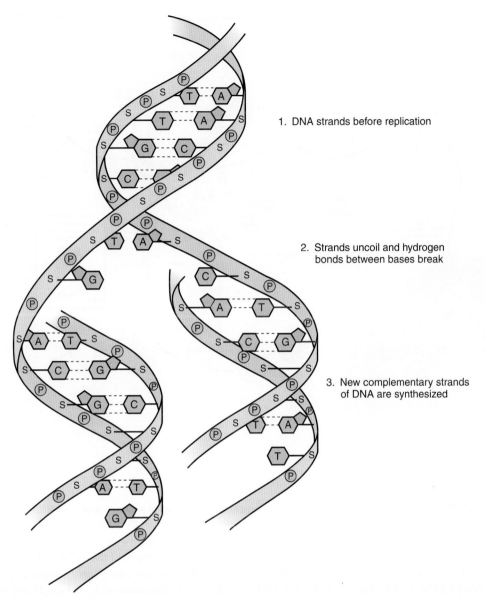

1. DNA strands before replication

2. Strands uncoil and hydrogen bonds between bases break

3. New complementary strands of DNA are synthesized

FIGURE 5.11   DNA replication. When a DNA molecule makes a copy of itself, it "unzips" to expose its nucleotide bases. Through the mechanism of obligatory base pairing, coordinated by the enzyme *DNA polymerase,* new DNA nucleotides bind to the exposed bases. This forms a new "other half" to each half of the original molecule. After all the bases have new nucleotides bound to them, two identical DNA molecules will be ready for distribution to the two daughter cells. (From Applegate: *The anatomy and physiology learning system,* ed 4, St Louis, 2011, Saunders.)

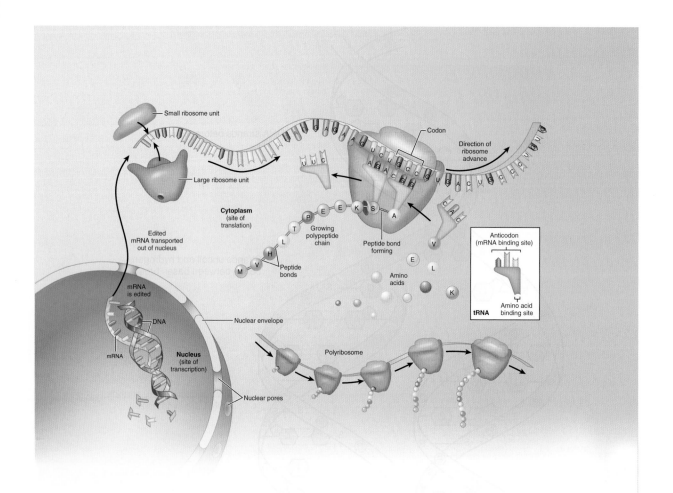

FIGURE 5.12   Protein synthesis begins with *transcription,* a process in which a messenger RNA (mRNA) molecule forms along one gene sequence of a DNA molecule within the cell's nucleus. As it is formed, the mRNA molecule separates from the DNA molecule, is edited, and leaves the nucleus through the large nuclear pores. Outside the nucleus, ribosome subunits attach to the beginning of the mRNA molecule and begin the process of *translation.* In translation, transfer RNA (tRNA) molecules bring specific amino acids—encoded by each mRNA codon—into place at the ribosome site. As the amino acids are brought into the proper sequence, they are joined together by peptide bonds to form long strands called *polypeptides.* Several polypeptide chains may be needed to make a complete protein molecule. (From Patton KT, Thibodeau GA: *Anatomy and physiology,* ed 9, St Louis, 2016, Mosby.)

REVIEW QUESTIONS

1. Which is the smallest classification within the biological hierarchy?
   A. Family
   B. Order
   C. Genus
   D. Species
2. Which statement is true regarding the scientific process?
   A. A scientific experiment must be repeatable.
   B. All scientists must follow the exact same steps.

C. The conclusion must support the hypothesis.
D. The experiment is the final step of the process.

3. Which term represents the amount of heat necessary to raise the temperature of 1 gram of a substance by 1° C?
   A. Specific heat
   B. Freezing point
   C. Boiling point
   D. Heat capacity

4. Which type of lipid is most commonly associated with the development of cardiovascular disease?
   A. Unsaturated fats
   B. Saturated fats
   C. Phospholipids
   D. Steroids

5. The liver performs most of the body's detoxification. Which organelle(s) should you expect to be present in large amounts in liver cells?
   A. Rough endoplasmic reticulum
   B. Smooth endoplasmic reticulum
   C. Bound ribosomes
   D. Free ribosomes

6. Which organelle converts food into energy to produce ATP?
   A. Lysosome
   B. Mitochondrion
   C. Nucleus
   D. Ribosome

7. Which term refers to a substance that speeds up a chemical reaction?
   A. Organelle
   B. Codon
   C. Enzyme
   D. Steroid

8. Bacterial cells reproduce by which process?
   A. Mitosis
   B. Meiosis
   C. Binary fission
   D. Cytokinesis

9. Which phase of cellular respiration takes place in both aerobic and anaerobic conditions?
   A. Electron transport chain
   B. Oxidative phosphorylation
   C. Krebs cycle
   D. Glycolysis

10. Which equation describes aerobic respiration?
    A. Glucose + Oxygen → Carbon dioxide + Water
    B. Glucose → Lactate + Energy
    C. Glucose → Carbon dioxide + Energy
    D. Carbon dioxide + Water → Glucose + Oxygen

11. Which are the end products of photosynthesis?
    A. Glucose and oxygen
    B. ATP and water
    C. NADH and oxygen
    D. Carbon dioxide and water

12. Which process occurs during interphase?
    A. Chromosomes align at the center of the cell.
    B. The nuclear envelope disappears.
    C. Chromosomes are duplicated.
    D. A parent cell separates into two daughter cells.

13. Which result occurs from variations in the way a gene is coded?
    A. Amino acid
    B. Codon
    C. Chromosome
    D. Allele

14. Which are the end results of meiosis?
    A. Two haploid daughter cells
    B. Four haploid daughter cells
    C. Two diploid daughter cells
    D. Four diploid daughter cells

15. Which is the first step of protein synthesis?
    A. Instructions in the DNA are copied onto mRNA.
    B. mRNA binds with ribosomes in the cytoplasm.
    C. tRNA carries amino acids to the ribosomal binding sites.
    D. Anticodons bind with complementary codons to form a base pair.

ANSWERS TO REVIEW QUESTIONS

1. D
2. A
3. A
4. B
5. B
6. B
7. C
8. C

9. D
10. A
11. A
12. C
13. D
14. B
15. A

6

CHEMISTRY

Chemistry is a part of our everyday lives. Almost three quarters of the objective information in a client's medical record consists of laboratory data derived from chemical analytical testing. Laboratory tests and chemical analysis play an important role in the detection, identification, and management of most diseases. The client's evaluation, diagnosis, treatment, care, and prognosis are, at least in part, based on the chemical information from laboratory tests that involve traditional technologies of chemistry. A sound, basic knowledge of chemistry enables the health care professional to reduce the risk of mishandled biologic samples and misdiagnosis and thereby deliver safer and higher quality care.

Chemistry is the study of matter and its properties. Everything in the universe is made or composed of different kinds of matter in one of its three states: solid, liquid, or gas. Matter is defined by its properties, and chemistry is a study of those properties and how those properties relate to one another. Chemistry is a very broad field of study and can be divided into many areas of specialization, such as physical or general chemistry, biochemistry, and organic and inorganic chemistry. This chapter reviews chemistry from the most basic of substances to very complex compounds.

CHAPTER OUTLINE

KEY TERMS

KEY TERMS—cont'd

Prefix	Ribose	Solute
Products	Scientific Notation	Solution
Proton	Significand	Solvent
Reactants	Single Replacement	Synthesis

Scientific Notation, The Metric System, and Temperature Scales

Scientific Notation

Scientific notation is the scientific system of writing numbers. Scientific notation is a method to write very big or very small numbers easily. Scientific notation is composed of three parts: a **mathematical sign** ($+$ or $-$), the **significand,** and the exponential, sometimes called the *logarithm.*

1. The mathematical sign designates whether the number is positive or negative.

HESI Hint

There is an understood ($+$) before a positive significand as there is in all positive numbers.

2. The significand is the base value of the number or the value of the number when all the values of ten are removed.
3. The exponential is a multiplier of the significand in powers of ten (Table 6.1). A positive exponential multiplies the significand by factors of ten. A negative exponential multiplies the significand by factors of one tenth (0.1).

HESI Hint

Some calculators or other devices may write the exponent as an "e" or "E" as in 3.2 e5 or 3.2 E5, called E notation, instead of 3.2×10^5, but it means the same.

Table 6.1 Exponentials*

10^9	1,000,000,000
10^6	1,000,000
10^3	1,000
10^2	100
10^1	10
10^0	1
10^{-2}	0.01
10^{-6}	0.000001
10^{-9}	0.000000001

*1.0 is understood to be the significand with each of the above exponentials.

Example

Consider -9.0462×10^5, where the minus ($-$) sign makes this a negative number, 9.0462 is the significand or base value, and 10^5 is the exponential or multiplier of the significand in the power of ten. In the example above, -9.0462×10^5 equals $-9.0462 \times 10 \times 10 \times 10 \times 10 \times 10$ or $-904,620$.

Example

Consider 4.7×10^{-3}, where the absence of the ($+$) sign is understood as positive, 4.7 is the significand or base value, and 10^{-3} is the exponential or multiplier of the significand in the negative power of ten (as tenths). In the example above, 4.7×10^{-3} equals ($4.7 \times 0.1 \times 0.1 \times 0.1$) or 0.0047.

HESI Hint

Move the decimal in the significand the number of places equal to the exponent of 10. When the exponent is positive, the decimal is moved to the right, and when the exponent is negative, the decimal is moved to the left.

HESI Hint

When writing a number between -1 and $+1$, always place a zero (0) to the left of the decimal. Write 0.62 and -0.39 (do not write .62 or $-.39$) to avoid mistakes when reading the number and locating the decimal.

The Metric System of Measurement

The metric system is a method to measure weight, length, and volume. It is a simple, logical, and efficient measurement system that is the standard in health professions. The basic measurements of the metric system are grams, liters, and meters. A gram (g) is the basic measure of weight, a liter (L) is the basic measure of volume, and a meter (m) is the basic measure of distance.

Each metric measurement is composed of a metric prefix and a basic unit of measure. An example is "kilogram," where "kilo" is the **prefix** and "gram" is the **basic unit of measure.** The prefixes have the same meaning or value, regardless of which basic unit of measurement (grams,

Table 6.2 The Prefixes

Prefix	Abbreviation	Means	Numerically
Tera	T-	10^{12}	1 trillion times
Giga	G-	10^{9}	1 billion times
Mega	M-	10^{6}	1 million times
Kilo	k-	10^{3}	1 thousand times
Hecto	h-	10^{2}	1 hundred times
Deka	D-	10^{1}	10 times
Deci	d-	10^{-1}	1 tenth of
Centi	c-	10^{-2}	1 hundredth of
Milli	m-	10^{-3}	1 thousandth of
Micro	μ-	10^{-6}	1 millionth of
Nano	n-	10^{-9}	1 billionth of
Pico	p-	10^{-12}	1 trillionth of
Femto	f-	10^{-15}	1 quadrillionth of

liters, or meters) is used. Prefixes are the quantifiers of the measurement units. All of the prefixes are based on multiples of ten. Any *one* of the prefixes can be combined with *one* of the basic units of measurement. Some examples are deciliter (dL), kilogram (kg), and millimeter (mm) (Table 6.2).

HESI Hint

Some comparisons may give more insight to sizes or amounts. A meter is a little more than 3 inches longer than a yard. A dime is a little less than 2 cm in diameter. A kilogram is about 2.2 lb. A liter is a little more than a quart.

Temperature Scales

The three most common temperature systems are **Fahrenheit, Celsius,** and **Kelvin.**

Fahrenheit (F) is a temperature measuring system used only in the United States, its territories, Belize, and Jamaica. It is rarely used for any scientific measurements except for body temperature (see Table 6.3). It has the following characteristics:
- Zero degrees (0° F) is the freezing point of sea water or heavy brine at sea level.
- 32° F is the freezing point of pure water at sea level.
- 212° F is the boiling point of pure water at sea level.
- Most people have a body temperature of 98.6° F.

Table 6.3 Important Temperatures in Fahrenheit and Celsius

Condition	Examples of Celsius (C) and Fahrenheit (F) Temperatures	
Freezing water	0° C	32° F
Normal body temperature	37° C	98.6° F
Boiling water	100° C	212° F

Celsius (sometimes called Centigrade) is a temperature system used in the rest of the world and by the scientific community. It has the following characteristics:
- Zero degrees (0° C) is the freezing point of pure water at sea level.
- 100° C is the boiling point of pure water at sea level.
- Most people have a body temperature of 37° C.

Kelvin (K) is used only in the scientific community. Kelvin has the following characteristics:
- Zero degrees (0K) is −273.15° C and is thought to be the lowest temperature achievable or absolute zero (0).
- The freezing point of water is 273K.
- The boiling point of water is 373K.
- Most people have a body temperature of 310K, but this is never used.

Atomic Structure and the Periodic Table

Atomic Structure

The basic building block of all molecules is the atom. An **atom's** physical structure is that of a **nucleus** and **orbits,** sometimes called **electron clouds.** The nucleus is at the center of the atom and is composed of **protons** and **neutrons.** At the outermost part of the atom are the orbits of the **electrons,** which spin around the nucleus at fantastic speeds, forming electron clouds. The speed of the electrons is so great that, in essence, they occupy the space around the nucleus as a cloud rather than as discrete individual locations. The electrons orbit the nucleus at various energy levels called *shells* or *orbits,* almost like the layers of an onion. As each orbital is filled to capacity, atoms begin adding electrons to the next orbit. An atom is most stable when its outermost orbit is full. However, most of the volume of an atom is empty space. See Figure 6.1 for examples of atoms.

Protons have a positive electrical charge, electrons have a negative charge, and neutrons have no charge at all. Ground state atoms tend to have equal numbers of protons and electrons, making them electrically neutral. When an atom is electrically charged, it is called an *ion* or it is said to be in an ionic state. This usually occurs when it is in a solution or in the form of a chemical compound. An atom in an ionic state will have lost electrons, resulting in a net positive charge, or will have gained electrons, resulting in a net negative charge. The atom is called a *cation* if it has a positive charge and an *anion* if it has a negative charge.

The Periodic Table

Matter is defined by its properties. It can also be stated that the properties of matter come from the properties of its composite elements, and the periodic table organizes the elements based on their structure and thus helps predict the properties of each of the elements (Fig. 6.2).

The **periodic table** is made up of a series of rows called **periods** (hence the name periodic table) and columns called **groups.** It is, at its simplest, a table of the known elements arranged according to their properties. The periodic table makes it possible to predict, for example, the charge of an atom or element, when it exists as an ion, by its location in the table. Group IA has a plus one (+1) charge, group IIA has a positive two (+2) charge, and group IIIA has a positive three (+3) charge. Group IVA can have either a positive four (+4) or a negative four (−4) charge. The negative charges are as follows: group VA has a negative three (−3) charge, group VIA has a negative two (−2) charge, and group VIIA has a negative one (−1) charge. Group VIIIA, called the noble gases, has no charge when in solution; it remains neutral in nearly all situations. Another property that can be generally deduced by the periodic chart is the number of electrons in the outer electron shell or cloud. Group IA will have one (1) electron in its outer shell. Group IIA will have two (2), Group IIIA will have three (3), Group IVA will have four (4), and on through all the A groups. Groups 3 IIIB through 12 IIB are called *transition metals* and are not as straightforward to predict because of some exceptions to the rules.

Atomic Number and Atomic Weight

Two important numbers or properties of atoms that can be obtained from the periodic table are the atomic number and the atomic mass.

The **atomic number** is the number of protons in the nucleus, and it defines an atom as a particular element. For instance, any atom that has

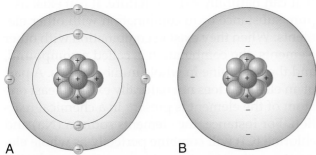

FIGURE 6.1   Models of the atom. The nucleus consists of protons (+) and neutrons at the core. Electrons inhabit outer regions called electron shells or energy levels **(A)** or **(B)** clouds. (From Patton KT, Thibodeau GA: *Anatomy and physiology,* ed 9, St Louis, 2016, Mosby.)

1 H 1.008																	2 He 4.002
3 Li 6.941	4 Be 9.012											5 B 10.811	6 C 12.011	7 N 14.007	8 O 15.999	9 F 18.998	10 Ne 20.180
11 Na 22.990	12 Mg 24.305											13 Al 26.982	14 Si 28.086	15 P 30.974	16 S 32.066	17 Cl 35.452	18 Ar 39.948
19 K 39.098	20 Ca 40.078	21 Sc 44.956	22 Ti 47.867	23 V 50.942	24 Cr 51.996	25 Mn 54.931	26 Fe 55.845	27 Co 58.933	28 Ni 58.963	29 Cu 63.546	30 Zn 65.39	31 Ga 69.723	32 Ge 72.61	33 As 74.922	34 Se 78.96	35 Br 79.904	36 Kr 83.80
37 Rb 85.468	38 Sr 87.62	39 Y 88.906	40 Zr 91.224	41 Nb 92.906	42 Mo 95.94	43 Tc (98)	44 Ru 101.07	45 Rh 102.906	46 Pd 106.42	47 Ag 107.868	48 Cd 112.411	49 In 114.818	50 Sn 118.710	51 Sb 121.760	52 Te 127.60	53 I 126.904	54 Xe 131.29
55 Cs 132.905	56 Ba 137.327	57 La 138.905	72 Hf 178.49	73 Ta 180.948	74 W 183.84	75 Re 186.207	76 Os 190.23	77 Ir 192.217	78 Pt 195.08	79 Au 196.967	80 Hg 200.59	81 Ti 204.383	82 Pb 207.2	83 Bi 208.980	84 Po (209)	85 At (210)	86 Rn (222)
87 Fr (223)	88 Ra 226.025	89 Ac 227.028	104 Rf (263.113)	105 Db (262.114)	106 Sg (266.122)	107 Bh (264.125)	108 Hs (269.134)	109 Mt (268.139)	110 Ds (272.146)	111 Rg (272.154)	112 Uub (277)	113 Uut (284)	114 Uuq (289)	115 Uup (288)	116 Uuh (292)	117 Uus (292)	118 Uuo (294)

Major elements
Trace elements

6
C
12.011 — Atomic number (number of protons) — Chemical symbol — Atomic weight (number of protons plus average number of neutrons)

58 Ce 140.115	59 Pr 140.907	60 Nd 144.24	61 Pm (145)	62 Sm 150.36	63 Eu 151.965	64 Gd 157.25	65 Eu 158.925	66 Gd 162.50	67 Ho 164.930	68 Er 167.26	69 Tm 168.939	70 Yb 173.04	71 Lu 174.967
90 Th 232.038	91 Pa 231.036	92 U 238.029	93 Np 237.048	94 Pu (244)	95 Am (243)	96 Cm (247)	97 Bk (247)	98 Cf (251)	99 Es (252)	100 Fm (257)	101 Md (258)	102 No (259)	103 Lr (260)

FIGURE 6.2 Periodic table of elements. (From Patton KT, Thibodeau GA: *Anatomy and physiology,* ed 9, St Louis, 2016, Mosby.)

eleven (11) protons, no matter how many neutrons or electrons, is sodium (Na). If an atom has six (6) protons, it is carbon (C). The atomic number is located at the top of each of the squares in a periodic table. It is always a whole number.

The **atomic weight** of an atom is the *average* mass of each of that element's **isotopes.** Isotopes are different kinds of the same atom that vary in weight. Protons and neutrons each have approximately the same mass or weight, which makes up nearly all of the atom's total mass. The atomic weight is the number at the bottom of each of the squares in the periodic table, and it is usually a decimal number. For a given element, the number of protons remains the same, whereas the number of neutrons varies to make the different isotopes. The combined number of protons and neutrons is the **mass number** of the element. The most common isotope of an atom, generally, has the same number of protons and neutrons in its nucleus. The element Carbon 12 (^{12}C), the most common carbon, has six (6) protons and six (6) neutrons. The isotope used for "carbon dating" is Carbon 14 (^{14}C), which has six (6) protons and eight (8) neutrons.

HESI Hint

The terms atomic weight and **atomic mass** are often used interchangeably, but they are not the same. Atomic mass is the mass of a *single atom*, whereas atomic weight is the weighted average of an atom and its isotopes. Atomic mass is *approximately* equal to mass number but is slightly larger because it takes into account all subatomic particles that contribute to the mass of an atom.

Chemical Equations

An element or atom is the simplest form of matter that can naturally exist in nature. It can exist as a pure substance or in combination with other elements. When they exist in combination with other elements, the combination is called a **compound,** and they combine in whole number ratios. A part of an element does not naturally exist; at least one atom of the element is present in a chemical reaction. For instance, the elements sodium (Na) and chlorine (Cl) will combine perfectly as whole elements or atoms in a one-to-one ratio to make the compound table salt (NaCl).

Chemical equations are simply recipes. Ingredients, called **reactants,** react to produce desired end results or compounds called **products.** Equations are written in the following manner:

Reactants → Products

In any chemical reaction, an arrow between the reactants and the products is present. This arrow symbolizes the direction of the reaction. Some reactions move toward the product side as seen above, and some reactions will move toward the reactant side with an arrow pointing toward the reactants instead of the products.

Reactants ← Products

There are also reactions that will create both reactants and products at the same time.

Reactants ↔ Products

An example is the reaction of aqueous silver nitrate ($AgNO_3$) and aqueous potassium chloride (KCl) to produce solid silver chloride (AgCl) and potassium nitrate (KNO_3).

$$AgNO_3 + KCl \rightarrow AgCl + KNO_3$$

Silver nitrate + potassium chloride yields
Silver chloride + potassium nitrate

The law of conservation of mass states that mass cannot be created or destroyed during a chemical reaction. Therefore, once the reactants have been written and the products predicted, the equation must be balanced. The same number of each element must be represented on both sides of the equation. The above example has one silver atom, one nitrogen atom, three oxygen atoms, one potassium atom, and one chloride atom on each side of the equation. Therefore, nothing in the way of matter was created or destroyed; it was simply rearranged.

Reaction Rates, Equilibrium, and Reversibility

Chemical reactions generally proceed at a specific rate. Some reactions are fast, and some are slow. A chemical reaction may proceed to completion, but some reactions may stop before all of the reactants are used to make products. These reactions are said to be at **equilibrium.** Equilibrium is a state in which reactants are forming products at the same rate that products are forming reactants. A reaction at equilibrium can be said to be reversible. As the chemicals A and B react to create C

and D, C and D react to make more A and B at the same rate.

$$A + B \leftrightarrow C + D$$

Through manipulation of the reaction by various means, shifts in equilibrium reversibility or the rate of the reaction can be controlled. There are basically four ways to increase the reaction rate: increase the temperature in the reaction, increase the surface area of the reactants, add a catalyst, or increase the concentrations of reactants.

Increasing the Temperature

Increasing the temperature causes the particles to have a greater kinetic energy, thereby causing them to move around faster, increasing their chances of contact and the energy with which they collide. Contact is when the chemical reactions occur.

Increasing the Surface Area

Increasing the surface area of the particles in the reaction gives the particles more opportunity to come into contact with one another. Wood shavings are an excellent example. One can increase the surface area of a log by cutting it into shavings or sawdust. Wood in the form of sawdust will burn or react much faster than a whole log.

Catalysts

A **catalyst** accelerates a reaction by reducing the activation energy or the amount of energy necessary for a reaction to occur. The catalyst is not used up in the reaction and can be collected at completion of the reaction. Various substances can be catalysts. Common examples include metals and proteins (protein catalysts are called enzymes).

Increasing the Concentration

Increasing the concentration of the reactants will cause more chance collisions between the reactants and produce more products. By analogy, if there are more cars on the road, there are likely to be more accidents or collisions. The more reactants there are, the faster and more often they will bump into each other and react or become products.

Solutions and Solution Concentrations

Solutions

A **solution** can be defined as a homogeneous mixture of two or more substances. In a solution, there is the **solute,** the part or parts that are being dissolved, and the **solvent,** the part that is doing the dissolving. Solutions can be a liquid in a liquid, a solid in a liquid, or a solid in a solid. The following are types of solutions.

- **Compounds:** Mixtures of different elements to create a single matter.
- **Alloys:** Solid solutions of metals to make a new one such as bronze, which is copper and tin, or steel, which is iron and carbon, and may contain tungsten, chromium, and manganese.
- **Amalgams**: A specific type of alloy in which a metal is dissolved in mercury.
- **Emulsions:** Mixtures of matter that readily separate such as water and oil.

Concentration of Solutions—Percent Concentration

Concentration is expressed as weight per weight, as in grams per grams; weight per volume, as in grams per liters; or volume per volume, as in milliliters per liter. Percent concentration is the expression of concentrations as parts per 100 parts. Therefore, most concentrations of this type are expressed as milligrams (mg) per 100 milliliters (mL), which can also be written as mg/100mL or mg/dL. A concentration expression of milliliters (mL) per 100 milliliters (mL) can be written as mL/100mL or mL/dL.

Concentration of Solutions—Molar Concentration

Molarity, or molar concentration, is a more sophisticated way to express concentrations than percent. One of the most important concepts in chemistry is the "mole." A **mole** is 6.02×10^{23} molecules of something. This number, 6.02×10^{23}, which is more than a trillion trillions, is known as *Avogadro's number*. A one molar solution will contain 6.02×10^{23} representative molecules of a solute in a liter of solvent. Molar concentrations are written as mol/L. It is important to note that if one measured the atomic mass of any element in grams (g), he or she will have weighed out one mole or 6.02×10^{23} atoms of that element or compound.

Chemical Reactions

A chemical reaction involves making or changing chemical bonds between elements or compounds to create new chemical compounds with different chemical formulas and different chemical properties. There are five main types of chemical reactions: synthesis, decomposition, combustion, single replacement, and double replacement. When a reaction occurs, the product is generally a molecule. A molecule may have a subscript written after the chemical symbol as in O_2, which is oxygen.

In a **synthesis** reaction, two elements combine to form a product. An example is the formation of potassium chloride salt when the element potassium (K^+) combines with the element chloride (Cl^-) in a solution:

$$2K^+ + 2Cl^- \rightarrow 2KCl$$

Two potassium atoms + two chloride atoms yields two molecules of potassium chloride.

Decomposition is often described as the opposite of synthesis because it is the breaking of a compound into its component parts.

$$NaCl \rightarrow Na^+ + Cl^-$$

When placed in an aqueous solution, table salt ($NaCl$) decomposes or breaks apart into an ionic solution of sodium (Na^+) as a cation and chloride (Cl^-) as an anion.

Combustion is a self-sustaining, exothermic (creates heat) chemical reaction where oxygen and a fuel compound such as a hydrocarbon react. In the combustion of hydrocarbon (gas or oil product), the products are carbon dioxide (CO_2) and water (H_2O). The combustion of ethane (C_2H_6) would look like this in a chemical equation, where (g) stands for gas:

$$2C_2H_6 \text{ (g)} + 7O_2 \text{ (g)} \rightarrow 4CO_2 \text{ (g)} + 6H_2O \text{ (g)}$$

Replacement reactions involve ionic compounds; whether or not the reaction will take place is based on the reactivity of the metals involved. **Single replacement** reactions consist of a more active metal reacting with an ionic compound containing a less active metal to produce a new compound. A good example is the reaction of copper (Cu) with aqueous silver nitrate ($AgNO_3$). The copper (Cu) and the silver (Ag) simply swap places. This type of reaction is referred to as single replacement and is illustrated in the following equation, where (aq) stands for aqueous and (s) stands for solid:

$$Cu\ (s) + 2AgNO_3\ (aq) \rightarrow Cu(NO_3)_2\ (aq) + 2Ag\ (s)$$

Copper + silver nitrate yields
copper nitrate + silver

Double replacement reactions involve two ionic compounds. The positive ion from one compound combines with the negative ion of the other compound. The result is two new ionic compounds that have "switched partners." The example of the reaction of silver nitrate ($AgNO_3$) and potassium chloride (KCl) is a good representation of double replacement:

$$AgNO_3 + KCl \rightarrow AgCl + KNO_3$$

Silver nitrate + potassium chloride yields
silver chloride + potassium nitrate

Chemical Bonding

Chemical bonding is the joining of one atom, element, or chemical to another. Some bonds are very weak, and some are nearly unbreakable. In many cases the type of bonding will be determined by the interplay of the electrons in the outer shell of the atom. There are two main types of chemical bonding: ionic and covalent.

An **ionic bond** is an electrostatic attraction between two oppositely charged ions, or a cation and an anion. This type of bond is generally formed between a metal and a nonmetal. An excellent example of ionic bonding is salt. Since opposites attract, the positive cation will attract the negative anion and form an electrostatic bond. In this type of a bond, the cation (sodium) *takes* one electron from the anion (chlorine), which makes the overall molecule electrically neutral. This *taking and giving* of an electron completes the outer electron orbits, making both substances very stable. Sodium (Na^+) needs one electron and Chlorine (Cl^-) has an extra one.

$$Na^+ + Cl^- \rightarrow NaCl$$

Sodium + chloride yields (table) salt

A **covalent bond** is formed when two atoms *share* electrons, generally in pairs, with one pair from each atom. A single covalent bond is the sharing of one pair of electrons. A double covalent bond is formed when two electron pairs are shared, and a triple covalent bond is formed when three electron pairs are shared. The covalent bond is the strongest of any type of chemical bond and is generally formed between two nonmetals (Fig. 6.3).

In a covalently bonded compound, if the electrons in the bond are shared equally, the bond is termed *non-polar*. However, not all elements share electrons equally within a bond. When this occurs, a polar bond is the result, which means that the shared electron density of the bond is concentrated around one atom more than the other. Polarity is based on the difference in electronegativity values for the elements involved in the bond. The greater the difference, the more polar the bond will be, or one end or side of the molecule will have a charge distinctly more positive and the other side of the molecule will be more negative in charge.

There are other types of attractions between particles called *intermolecular forces*. These are not bonding interactions between atoms within a

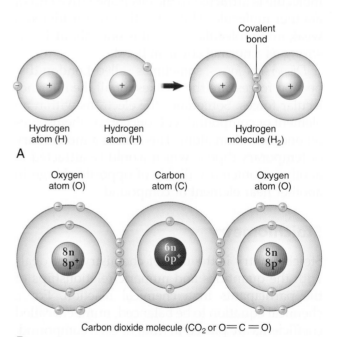

Carbon dioxide molecule (CO_2 or $O = C = O$)

FIGURE 6.3 Types of covalent bonds. **A,** A single covalent bond forms by the sharing of one electron pair between two atoms of hydrogen, resulting in a molecule of hydrogen gas. **B,** A double covalent bond (double bond) forms by the sharing of two pairs of electrons between two atoms. In this case, two double bonds form: one between carbon and each of the two oxygen atoms. (From Patton KT, Thibodeau GA: *Anatomy and physiology,* ed 9, St Louis, 2016, Mosby.)

molecule but instead are weaker forces of attraction between whole molecules. These forces are hydrogen bonding, dipole-dipole interactions, and dispersion forces.

A *hydrogen bond* is the attraction for a hydrogen atom by a highly electronegative element. The elements generally involved are fluorine (F), oxygen (O), and nitrogen (N). Hydrogen bonds are about 5% to 10% as strong as covalent bonds, making them the strongest of the intermolecular forces.

A *dipole-dipole interaction* is the attraction of one dipole on one molecule for the dipole of another molecule. A dipole is created when an electron pair is shared unequally in a covalent bond between two atoms or elements (discussed earlier in polar covalent bonding). Because the electrons are shared unequally, the molecule, not the covalent bond, will have a positive end and a negative end or side. In a solution, the molecules will align the charged ends of the molecule north to south or positive to negative, where the north end on one molecule is next to the south end of another. The result is a weak bond between molecules, where the more highly electropositive end of a molecule is attracted to the electronegative end of another molecule. This attraction is considered a weak intermolecular force. It is only about 1% as strong as a normal covalent bond.

Dispersion forces, sometimes called London dispersion forces, are the weakest of all the intermolecular forces. Sometimes the electrons within an element or compound will concentrate themselves on one side of an atom. This causes a momentary or temporary dipole, which would be attracted to another momentary dipole of opposite charge in another near element or compound.

Stoichiometry

Stoichiometry is the part of chemistry that deals with the quantities and numeric relationships of the participants in a chemical reaction. For a chemical equation to be balanced, numbers called coefficients are placed in front of each compound. These numbers are used in a ratio to compare how much of one substance is needed to react with another in a certain reaction. The process is similar to comparing ingredients in a recipe.

$$2C_2H_6 + 7O_2 \rightarrow 4CO_2 + 6H_2O$$

Ethane + oxygen yields carbon dioxide + water

Using this reaction, determine the number of moles of oxygen (O_2) that will react with four (4) moles of ethane (C_2H_6). It is possible to determine the number of moles of oxygen needed to complete the reaction using a process called *dimensional analysis*:

$$\frac{4 \text{ mol } C_2H_6}{} \left| \frac{7 \text{ mol } O_2}{2 \text{ mol } C_2H_6} \right. = 14 \text{ mol } O_2$$

By multiplying the given amount of four moles of ethane by the actual amount of seven moles of oxygen (O_2) and dividing by the actual number of two moles of ethane (C_2H_6), one can determine that the number of moles of oxygen needed to react will be fourteen.

Oxidation and Reduction

Oxidation/reduction reactions, called *redox*, involve the transfer of electrons from one element to another. *Oxidation is the loss of electrons, and reduction is the gain of electrons.* It is not possible to have one without the other. The element that is oxidized (loses electron) is the reductant or reducing agent, and the element that is reduced (gains electron) is the oxidant or the oxidizing agent. Even though a substance is oxidized and gains an electron, its ionic charge is more negative; likewise, a substance that is reduced loses an electron, and its ionic charge is more positive.

HESI Hint

A good mnemonic is "OIL-RIG" or Oxidation Is Loss (of an electron), Reduction Is Gain (of an electron). Think of it this way: to "reduce" an element, one must cause that element's overall electrical charge to become less, and that is done by adding or gaining one or more negatively charged electrons ($e-$).

A Redox Reaction

Oxidant (gains electron) + e^- $\leftrightarrow$ Reductant (loses electron) – e^-
      Reduced   Oxidized

The oxidant is reduced because it gains an electron. The reductant is oxidized because it loses an electron.

To identify what has been oxidized and what has been reduced, the oxidation states of all elements in the compound must be determined. The following is a series of rules to make those determinations:

1. The oxidation number of any elemental atom is zero. This means that if an element is in its *natural* state, its charge or number is zero. Most elements in their standard states are single atoms. However, a few exceptions exist including hydrogen (H_2), bromine (Br_2), oxygen (O_2), nitrogen (N_2), iodine (I_2), and fluorine (F_2). When these elements exist outside of a compound in their natural state, they are always in pairs.
2. The oxidation number of any simple ion is the charge of the ion. If in a reaction, sodium (Na) was listed as an ion (Na^+), it would have an oxidation number of plus one ($+1$). If chlorine (Cl) was listed as an ion (Cl^-), it would have an oxidation number of minus one (-1).
3. The oxidation number for oxygen in a compound is minus two (-2).
4. The oxidation number for hydrogen in a compound is plus one ($+1$).
5. The sum of the oxidation numbers equals the charge on the molecules or polyatomic ions.

Example: Assign oxidation numbers to all elements in the following reactions.

$$2C_2H_6 + 7O_2 \rightarrow 4CO_2 + 6H_2O$$

Ethane + oxygen yields carbon dioxide + water

By using the rules listed earlier, we can use simple algebra to solve for the change of electrical charges of those elements not discussed in the rules. In solving for carbon, the first element in the first reactant, ethane (C_2H_6), we can ignore the coefficient because it has nothing to do with the oxidation states of any of the elements. The total charge on the compound is zero, as is determined using rule five. From rule four, hydrogen must have an oxidation state of $+1$. There are six hydrogen molecules, so the total charge of the hydrogen molecules is $+6$. Following is the algebra to solve for the oxidation state of carbon (x):

$$2x + 6 (+1) = 0$$

Solving for *x*, carbon is found to have a charge of -3.

If the same method is used, the states of all the other elements can be determined. Oxygen in O_2 is zero (rule one). Carbon in CO_2 is $+4$, and oxygen is -2. Finally, hydrogen in water is $+1$, and oxygen is -2. With this information, it is possible to predict what is oxidized and what is reduced. Look at the charges on either side of the equation and see what has changed. Carbon goes from a state of -3 to a state of $+4$. It has lost seven electrons and has, therefore, been oxidized. Oxygen's state has changed from 0 to -2. It has gained two electrons and has, therefore, been reduced.

Acids and Bases

Acids are corrosive to metals; they change blue litmus paper red and become less acidic when mixed with bases. **Bases,** also called *alkaline compounds,* are substances that denature proteins, making them feel very slick; they change red litmus paper blue and become less basic when mixed with acids.

Acids are compounds that are hydrogen or proton donors. *Hydrogen in its ionic state is simply a proton.* In water, naked protons exist only for a short time before reacting with other water molecules to produce H_3O^+, a substance called hydronium. Hydronium is a water molecule plus a proton or hydrogen.

Bases are hydrogen or proton acceptors and generally have a hydroxide (OH) group in the makeup of the molecule. This definition explains the dissociation of water into low concentrations of hydronium and hydroxide ions:

$$H_2O + H_2O \leftrightarrow H_3O^+ + OH^-$$

Water + water yields acid + base

In this example, one water (H_2O) molecule acts as a hydrogen donor, giving one of its two hydrogens to another water molecule and in the process producing the hydronium (H_3O^+) cation and leaving a hydroxyl group (OH). All acids produce hydronium when placed in H_2O. As can be seen, H_2O is amphoteric, which means it can act as both an acid and a base. In the example above, one molecule of H2O acts as the proton donor, becoming a hydroxide (OH), and another molecule acts as the proton acceptor, becoming the conjugate acid (H_3O^+).

The concentration of acids is expressed as **pH.** The pH scale commonly in use ranges from 0 to 14 and is a measure of the acidity or alkalinity of a solution (Fig. 6.4). A neutral solution that is neither acidic nor basic has a value of 7. Lower numbers mean more acidic, and higher numbers mean more basic.

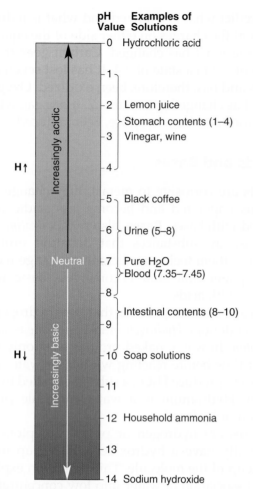

pH Value   **Examples of Solutions**

Increasingly acidic

H↑

Neutral

Increasingly basic

H↓

- 0 Hydrochloric acid
- 1
- 2 Lemon juice
- Stomach contents (1–4)
- 3 Vinegar, wine
- 4
- 5 Black coffee
- 6 Urine (5–8)
- 7 Pure H₂O
- Blood (7.35–7.45)
- 8
- Intestinal contents (8–10)
- 9
- 10 Soap solutions
- 11
- 12 Household ammonia
- 13
- 14 Sodium hydroxide

FIGURE 6.4   The pH range. (From Herlihy: The human body in health and illness, ed 5, St Louis, 2014, Saunders.)

Nuclear Chemistry

Chemical and nuclear reactions are quite different. In chemical reactions, atoms are trying to reach stable electron configurations. Nuclear chemistry is concerned with reactions that take place in the nucleus to obtain stable nuclear configurations. *Radioactivity* is the word used to describe the emission of particles and/or energy from an unstable nucleus. The particles and/or energy that are emitted are referred to as *radiation*. The three types of radiation in nuclear chemistry are alpha, beta, and gamma.

Alpha radiation is the emission of helium nuclei. These particles contain two protons and two neutrons, causing them to have a charge of plus two (+2). Alpha particles are the largest of the radioactive emissions, and penetration from alpha particles can generally be stopped by a piece of paper.

Beta radiation is a product of the decomposition of a neutron or proton. It is actually composed of high-energy, high-speed electrons that began as neutrons or protons. These particles are either negatively charged (electrons) or positively charged (positrons). Because they have virtually no mass, beta particles can be stopped by a thin sheet of aluminum foil, Lucite, or plastic.

Gamma radiation is high-energy electromagnetic radiation, similar to x-rays but with more energy. It is very penetrating and can go through several feet of concrete or several inches of lead. Lead shielding is required to block gamma rays.

An isotope is written as an abbreviation with the symbol of the element preceded by a superscript number indicating the atomic mass. For example, Iodine-131 is correctly abbreviated as ^{131}I, and Iodine-125 would be written as ^{125}I. In nature, some isotopes are stable and some are unstable. Given enough time, unstable nuclei will change or "decay" into more stable forms. The amount of time it takes for half of the unstable isotope to decay is called the half-life. In nuclear chemistry, the unstable atom *decays* until it finds a stable nuclear configuration, usually by emitting radioactive particles. The amount of time used in a half-life ($T^{1/2}$) is different for every radioactive element. Some half-lives are very long, and some are as short as a few days. An example of radioactive half-life or decay is ^{131}I, which has a half-life of approximately 8 days, or every 8 days one-half of the radioactive particles will be emitted or decayed. This will happen over and over again until the ^{131}I reaches a stable nuclear configuration.

Biochemistry

Biochemistry is the study of chemical processes in living organisms. Much of biochemistry deals with the structures and functions of molecules such as carbohydrates, proteins, lipids, and nucleic acids.

Carbohydrates

Sugars and starches are carbohydrates. Their most important function is to store and provide energy for the body. The sugars **deoxyribose** and **ribose** are used in the formation of deoxyribonucleic acid (DNA) and ribonucleic acid (RNA), respectively. Carbohydrates are more abundant than any other known type of biomolecule.

The simplest type of carbohydrate is a **monosaccharide**. Monosaccharides contain carbon,

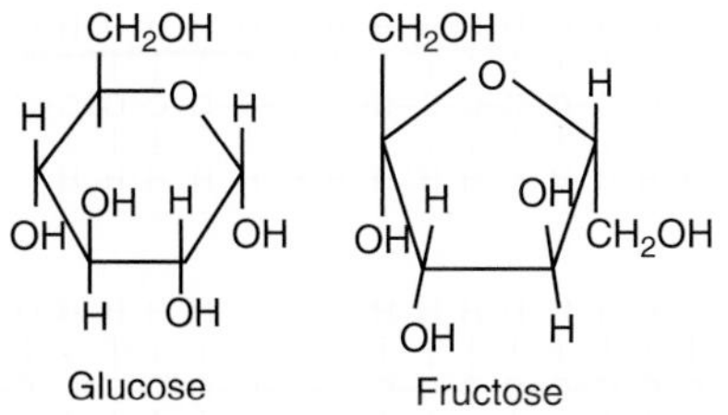

FIGURE 6.5 Molecular configuration for glucose and fructose.

hydrogen, and oxygen in a ratio of 1:2:1 (general formula $C_m(H_2O)_n$, where m is at least three). Glucose ($C_6H_{12}O_6$) is one of the most important carbohydrates and is an example of a monosaccharide. Fructose ($C_6H_{12}O_6$), the sugar commonly associated with the sweet taste of fruits, is also a monosaccharide. Glucose and fructose are both a six-carbon sugar called a *hexose* (Fig. 6.5).

HESI Hint

The word "saccharide" comes from a Greek word meaning "sugar."

HESI Hint

Glucose and fructose have the same chemical formula ($C_6H_{12}O_6$) but different actual molecular configurations.

Two monosaccharides can be joined together to make a **disaccharide**. The most well-known disaccharide is sucrose, which is ordinary sugar. Sucrose consists of a glucose molecule and a fructose molecule joined together. Another disaccharide is lactose, or milk sugar, consisting of a glucose molecule and a galactose molecule. Figure 6.6 illustrates the molecular configuration of sucrose and lactose.

When three to six monosaccharides are joined together, it is called an *oligosaccharide* (oligo meaning "few"). More than six and up to thousands of monosaccharides joined together make a *polysaccharide,* which can be called a *starch.* Two of the most common polysaccharides are cellulose,

made by plants, and glycogen, made by animals; both of these polysaccharides are chains of repeating glucose units.

Carbohydrates as Energy

Glycolysis Glucose is mainly metabolized by a chemical pathway in the body called glycolysis. The net result is the breakdown of one molecule of glucose into two molecules of pyruvate; this also produces a net two molecules of adenosine triphosphate (ATP). ATP is the substance cells use for energy. In aerobic cells with sufficient oxygen, like most human cells, the pyruvate is further metabolized by a process called *oxidative phosphorylation* (Krebs cycle) generating more molecules of ATP, water, and carbon dioxide. Using oxygen to completely oxidize glucose provides an organism with far more energy than any oxygen-deficient system.

When skeletal muscles are used in vigorous exercise, they will not have enough oxygen to meet their energy demands. They will need to use another type of glucose metabolism called anaerobic glycolysis. Anaerobic means in the absence of or without oxygen. This process converts glucose to lactate instead of pyruvate as in aerobic glycolysis. The production of lactate, an acid, in the muscles creates the "burning or cramping" sensation during intense exercise.

HESI Hint

An aerobic organism or cell requires oxygen to sustain life. An anaerobic organism or cell can function in low concentrations of oxygen, also called micro-aerobic, and some anaerobic organisms exist with no oxygen present.

Gluconeogenesis The liver can make glucose from other noncarbohydrate sources, such as proteins and parts of fats, using a process called gluconeogenesis. The glucose produced can then enter the energy-producing cycles mentioned

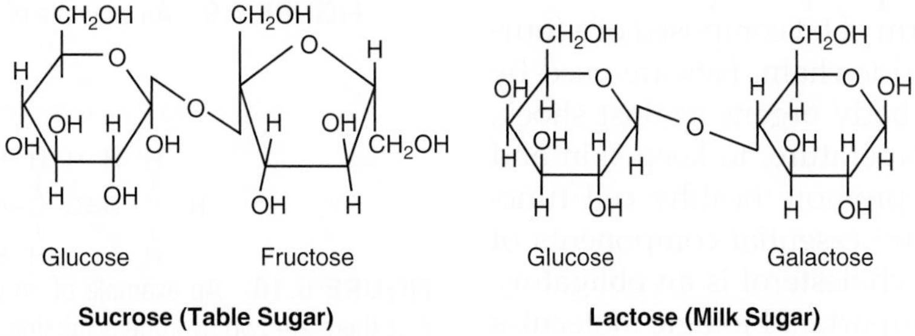

Sucrose (Table Sugar)   **Lactose (Milk Sugar)**

FIGURE 6.6 Molecular configuration for sucrose and lactose.

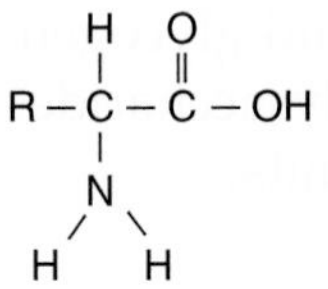

$$R - \overset{\overset{\displaystyle H}{|}}{\underset{\underset{\displaystyle N}{|}}{C}} - \overset{\overset{\displaystyle O}{\|}}{C} - OH$$

FIGURE 6.7   An amino acid general formula.

previously and undergo glycolysis, or glucose can be stored as glycogen in animals or as cellulose in plants. Glucose can also be used to make other saccharides.

Proteins

Proteins are made up of amino acids. An amino acid is a molecule composed of a carbon atom bonded with four other groups: an amine group (NH2), a carboxyl group (COOH), a hydrogen, and an R group (Fig. 6.7). The R group is different for each amino acid, giving each amino acid its own identity and characteristics. Amino acids are joined together to make proteins or parts of proteins. A union of two amino acids using a peptide bond is called a *dipeptide;* groups of fewer than 30 amino acids are called peptides or polypeptides. Larger groups are referred to as proteins. As an example, an important protein in blood called *albumin* contains 585 amino acid residues, and albumin is considered a fairly small protein. In humans, there are only 20 amino acids needed to make all the proteins necessary for life.

Lipids

Lipids are fats and encompass a large group of molecules, including oils, fats, and fatty acids. Fatty acids consist of a hydrocarbon chain with an acid group, the carboxyl group (COOH), at one end. A neutral fat (triglyceride) is three fatty acids generally joined to a glycerol or some other backbone structure (Fig. 6.8). Phospholipids are similar to neutral fats, but one of the three fatty acids is replaced by a phosphate group. Cholesterol is yet another form of fat composed of a four-ring structure and a side chain. Fats are used by the body to insulate body organs against shock, to maintain body temperature, to keep skin and hair healthy, and to promote healthy cell function. Phospholipids are essential components of cell membranes, and cholesterol is an obligatory precursor for many important biologic molecules such as steroid hormones. Fats also serve as energy stores for the body.

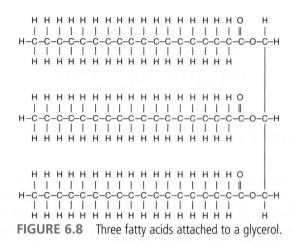

FIGURE 6.8   Three fatty acids attached to a glycerol.

Lipids are found in many foods, such as oils, milk, and milk products such as butter and cheese. Natural lipids can be classified as unsaturated, polyunsaturated, and saturated. Saturated fats have no double bond between carbon atoms of the fatty acid chains (Fig. 6.9). Unsaturated fats have one or more double bonds between some of the carbon atoms of the fatty acid chains and are more desirable in our diet than saturated fats (Fig. 6.10).

Nucleic Acids

Nucleic acids are the biologic brain of life, telling the cell what it will do and how to do it. They include DNA and RNA. Both are nucleotide chains that convey genetic information. Nucleic acids are found in all living cells and viruses. Most nucleic acids are found in the nucleus, but some are found in the cytoplasm and mitochondria of individual cells. They are very large molecules that have two main parts.

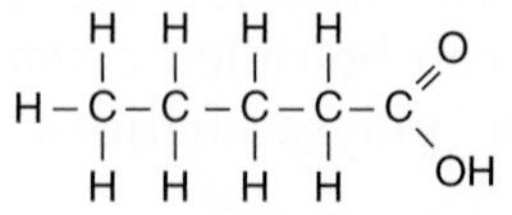

FIGURE 6.9   An example of a saturated fatty acid.

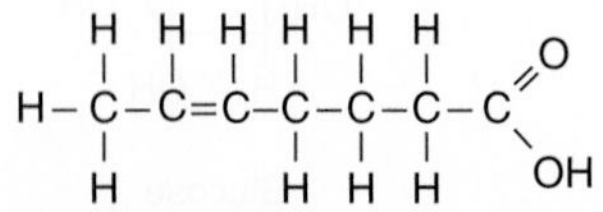

FIGURE 6.10   An example of an unsaturated fatty acid. Note that there are two hydrogens missing, and there is a double bond, designated by two lines, between the two carbons in the center of the fatty acid.

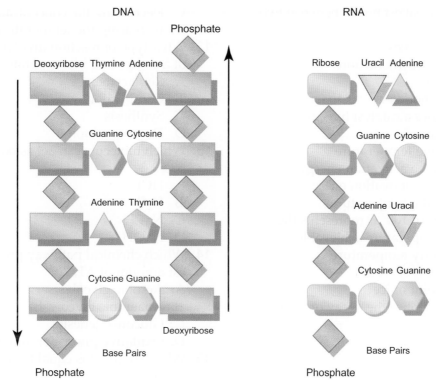

FIGURE 6.11 Structure of DNA and RNA. (Note: The double helix is not illustrated here.)

The backbone of the molecule DNA is composed of deoxyribose, a five-carbon sugar that is also called a pentose, and a phosphate, which alternately chain together in a "sugar-phosphate-sugar-phosphate" chain, making two very long structures. The two chains, or strands, actually twist around each other like the strands of a rope, which is referred to as a "double helix."

The DNA bases adenine, cytosine, guanine, and thymine join the two chains from sugar to sugar much like the rungs of a ladder in a base pair relationship. The pair relationships are constant in that adenine and thymine are always bound together and cytosine and guanine are always bound together in DNA. Note that the two sugar-phosphate chains in DNA run in opposite directions: one up and one down. This is termed *anti-parallel*.

The structure of RNA differs from DNA's structure in that RNA is a single strand of ribose, a five-carbon carbohydrate, in a sugar-phosphate chain (Fig. 6.11). RNA does not use thymine to form one of its base pairs; it uses instead uracil to bind with adenine. Cytosine and guanine are the other base pair.

REVIEW QUESTIONS

1. An individual who weighs 70 kg weighs how many pounds?
   A. 154 lbs
   B. 140 lbs
   C. 35 lbs
   D. 32 lbs
2. How many protons does oxygen (O) have? Refer to the periodic table.
   A. 24
   B. 16
   C. 8
   D. 6
3. The atomic number of an atom is equal to the number of:
   A. Electrons
   B. Neutrons
   C. Protons
   D. Isotopes
4. Oxidation refers to the:
   A. Loss of electrons
   B. Sharing of electrons
   C. Gaining of electrons
   D. Unsharing of electrons

5. What are the weakest bonds between two molecules?
    A. Dispersion forces
    B. Dipole-dipole interactions
    C. Ionic bonds
    D. Hydrogen bonds
6. What effect does a catalyst have on a chemical reaction?
    A. Increases the temperature
    B. Decreases the activation energy
    C. Increases the activation energy
    D. Decreases the temperature
7. A temperature of $100°$ C represents the:
    A. Highest temperature achievable
    B. Normal body temperature
    C. Boiling point of water
    D. Melting point of ice
8. What term describes the decay of an unstable isotope?
    A. Half-life
    B. Decomposition
    C. Sublimation
    D. Reduction
9. Which of the following is an example of a double replacement reaction?
    A. $NaCl \rightarrow Na^+ + Cl^-$
    B. $Cl_2 + H_2O \rightarrow HOCl + HCl$
    C. $2Na + 2HCl \rightarrow 2NaCl + H_2$
    D. $2C_2H_6 + 7O_2 \rightarrow 4CO_2 + 6H_2O$
10. What is the correct coefficient for the products of the following reaction when the equation is balanced? $C_6H_{12}O_6 + 6O_2 \rightarrow \_CO_2 + \_H_2O$
    A. 2
    B. 4
    C. 6
    D. 8
11. Which of the following increases the rate of a chemical reaction?
    A. Increasing the activation energy
    B. Decreasing the surface area

C. Decreasing the concentration
D. Increasing the temperature
12. What type of reaction involves the breaking of a compound into separate components?
    A. Replacement
    B. Combustion
    C. Synthesis
    D. Decomposition
13. Which molecule can act as both an acid and a base?
    A. HCl
    B. H_2O
    C. NaCl
    D. NaOH
14. Which chemical pathway produces the greatest amount of ATP?
    A. Aerobic glycolysis
    B. Anaerobic glycolysis
    C. Gluconeogenesis
    D. Oxidative phosphorylation
15. What exponent is equal to 10,000?
    A. 10^6
    B. 10^5
    C. 10^4
    D. 10^3
16. What macromolecules are responsible for passing on genetic information?
    A. Proteins
    B. Nucleic acids
    C. Carbohydrates
    D. Lipids
17. Which term refers to a large group of amino acids joined together?
    A. Protein
    B. Dipeptide
    C. Peptide
    D. Polypeptide

ANSWERS TO REVIEW QUESTIONS

1. A
2. C
3. C
4. A
5. A
6. B
7. C
8. A
9. B

10. C
11. D
12. D
13. B
14. D
15. C
16. B
17. D

ANATOMY AND PHYSIOLOGY

7

From cells and tissues to organs and systems, the human body is one of the most complex organisms on earth. Members of health professions who take care of patients need to know how the human body works as a whole, and what role specific parts of the body play in an individual's health and well-being. This information is the basis of understanding conditions, diseases, and dysfunctions, and what methods are appropriate to use for patients experiencing these.

A 1-year course in anatomy and physiology should be undertaken before the student prepares for the anatomy and physiology examination. Additionally, taking time to study anatomy and physiology at every opportunity is excellent preparation. This guide discusses each of the major body systems and emphasizes the most important information to know.

CHAPTER OUTLINE

General Terminology	Muscular System	Urinary System
Cytology	Nervous System	Reproductive System
Mitosis and Meiosis	Endocrine System	Review Questions
Histology	Cardiovascular System	Answers to Review Questions
Integumentary System	Respiratory System	
Skeletal System	Digestive System	

KEY TERMS

Anatomic Position	Epidermis	Neurons
Anterior	Erythrocytes	Organelle
Appendicular Skeleton	External Respiration	Osteoblasts
Autonomic Nervous System	Hemopoiesis	Osteoclasts
Axial Skeleton	Histology	Planes
Brainstem	Inferior	Posterior
Cell	Internal Respiration	Proximal
Cerebellum	Lateral	Sarcomeres
Cerebrum	Leukocytes	Sliding Filament Model
Cytology	Medial	Superficial
Deep	Meiosis	Superior
Dermis	Mitosis	Thrombocytes
Diencephalon	Nephrons	
Distal	Neuroglia	

General Terminology

Standard terminology is used across all health professions to facilitate common understanding. This terminology includes directions for locating structures on and within the body, as well as for subdivisions and regions of the body.

Anatomic position provides a baseline reference point for areas of the body. In this position, the body is erect, the feet are slightly apart, the head is held high, the arms are at the sides, and the palms of the hands are facing forward.

Planes are imaginary flat plates. A section is a real or virtual cut made along a plane. A sagittal plane divides the body or body part into right and left sides. A midsagittal plane divides the body into equal right and left halves. A frontal (coronal) plane divides the body or body part into front (anterior) to back (posterior) sections. A transverse (horizontal) plane divides the body or body part into upper (superior) and lower (inferior) sections.

Directional terms to review include **superior** (above), **inferior** (below), **anterior** (toward the front), **posterior** (toward the back), **medial** (toward the midline), and **lateral** (away from the midline). **Proximal** and **distal** are terms of direction and are used in reference to the extremities. Proximal means closer to the point of attachment of the extremity to the trunk, and distal refers to farther away from the point of attachment of the extremity to the trunk. Figure 7.1 depicts planes and directional terms. Additionally, **superficial** means closer to or at the surface of the body, and **deep** means further into the body.

Major body cavities are divided into the dorsal cavity, which includes the cranial and spinal cavities, and the ventral cavity, which includes the thoracic and abdominopelvic cavities.

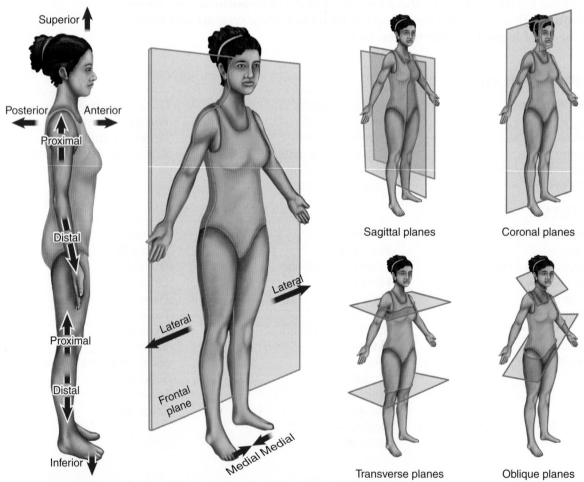

FIGURE 7.1   Planes and directions of the body. (From Patton KT, Thibodeau GA: *Anatomy and physiology*, ed 9, St Louis, 2016, Mosby.)

Additional useful terminology is defined later in this chapter.

Cytology

Cytology is the study of cells. The **cell** is the basic unit of life, and the building block of tissues and organs. The major parts of the cell are the plasma membrane, cytoplasm, nucleus, and organelles. The nucleus contains deoxyribonucleic acid (DNA) which is genetic material that codes for proteins. Proteins are major components of body structures and are part of enzymes and hormones which regulate all chemical reactions within the body. Each **organelle** has a specific function.

Ribosomes synthesize proteins. Rough endoplasmic reticulum (ER) has ribosomes for synthesizing proteins; smooth ER synthesizes lipids and carbohydrates. Golgi apparatus packages substances from the ER. Mitochondria synthesize adenosine triphosphate, i.e., ATP, which is the body's energy molecule. Lysosomes digests molecules such as pathogens and worn out cell parts. Centrioles organize and move chromosomes during cell reproduction. Cilia are extensions that move substances over the surface of the cell.

Mitosis and Meiosis

Mitosis is necessary for growth and repair. In this process of cell division, the DNA is duplicated and distributed evenly to two identical daughter cells. **Meiosis** is the special cell division that takes place in the gonads, which are the ovaries and testes. In this process, the number of chromosomes is reduced from 46 to 23, so that when the egg and the sperm unite in fertilization, the zygote will have the correct number of chromosomes.

Histology

Histology is the study of tissues. A tissue is a group of cells that act together to perform specific functions. The four types of tissues are epithelial, connective, muscle, and nervous (Fig. 7.2). Epithelial tissue covers, lines, and protects the body and its internal organs. Glandular epithelium secretes substances such as mucus, enzymes, and

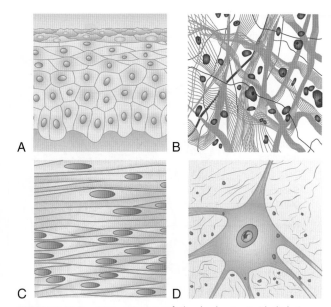

FIGURE 7.2 Major tissues of the body. **A,** Epithelial tissue; **B,** connective tissue; **C,** muscle tissue; **D,** nervous tissue. (From Patton KT, Thibodeau GA: *Anatomy and physiology,* ed 9, St Louis, 2016, Mosby.)

hormones. Connective tissue is the most abundant tissue in the body. It forms the framework of the body, providing support and structure for the organs. Types include fibrous (areolar, adipose, reticular, dense), bone, cartilage, and blood.

Nervous tissue is composed of **neurons**, which initiate and conduct nerve impulses, and connective tissue cells called **neuroglia**, which support the neurons. Muscle tissue has the ability to contract or shorten, as well as to lengthen. Muscle tissue is classified as voluntary (skeletal muscles) or involuntary (smooth muscle and cardiac muscle tissue).

Integumentary System

The integumentary system consists of the skin and its structures and organs such as hair, nails, and sensory receptors. The skin is the largest organ of the body. Its structure is illustrated in Figure 7.3. The two layers of the skin are the **epidermis**, the outermost protective layer made of dead, keratinized epithelial cells, and the **dermis**, the underlying layer of connective tissue with blood vessels, nerve endings, and the associated skin structures. The dermis rests on subcutaneous tissue, also known as hypodermis or superficial fascia, which connects the skin to underlying muscles and bones.

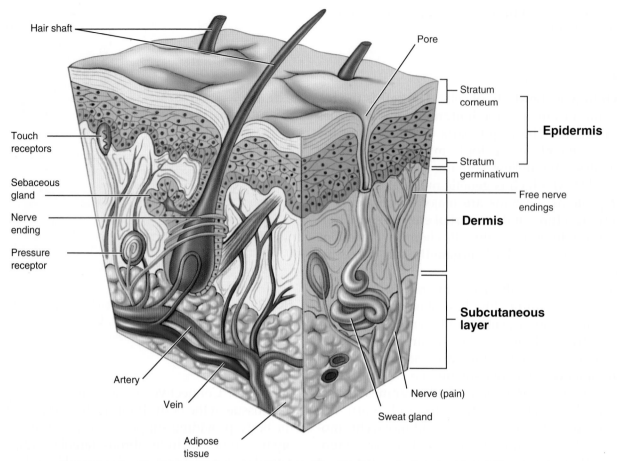

FIGURE 7.3 Diagram of skin structure. (From Herlihy: *The human body in health and illness,* ed 5, St Louis, 2014, Saunders.)

The layers of the epidermis from superficial to deep are the stratum corneum, stratum lucidum, stratum granulosum, stratum spinosum, and stratum germinativum (stratum basale), which continually undergoes mitosis. Epidermal cells contain *keratin,* which waterproofs the skin, and melanocytes produce the pigment *melanin,* which darkens the skin to protect against radiation from the sun.

The dermis is composed of fibrous connective tissue and contains blood vessels, sensory nerve endings, hair follicles, and glands. There are two types of sweat glands. Eccrine sweat glands are the most widely distributed and regulate body temperature by releasing a watery secretion that evaporates from the surface of the skin. Apocrine sweat glands are mainly found in the axilla and inguinal regions. This sweat is thicker because it contains bits of cytoplasm from the secreting cells. This cell debris attracts bacteria, and the presence of the bacteria on the skin results in body odor.

Sebaceous glands release an oily secretion called sebum through hair follicles; it lubricates the skin and prevents drying. These glands are susceptible to becoming clogged and attracting bacteria, particularly during adolescence, resulting in acne. The appendages of the skin include hair and nails. Both are composed of plates of keratin. Hair, nails, and skin may show changes in disease that may be used in the diagnosis of clinical conditions. For example, melanoma is a cancer associated with the skin. Blue-tinged nails can indicate lack of adequate blood oxygenation. Thin, brittle hair may indicate malnutrition.

HESI Hint

As the epidermal cells move from the deepest layers to the superficial layers, they move away from their blood and nutrient supply; subsequently, they dehydrate and die. To illustrate this, visualize a large transparent container filled with inflated balloons covered with sticky glue. This illustrates the stratum basale. As the balloons deflate, the sides that are stuck together pull the balloons into a spiny shape, much like the stratum spinosum. As the balloons continue to deflate, they become flattened, like the stratum corneum.

Skeletal System

The body framework consists of bone, cartilage, ligaments, and joints. Functions of the skeletal system include support, movement, blood cell formation (**hemopoiesis**), protection of internal organs, provision of muscle attachment sites, and mineral storage, especially calcium and phosphorus.

The two types of bone tissue are compact (dense) and spongy (cancellous). Compact bone forms the outer layer of all bones. Spongy bone contains a latticework of plates of bone with spaces in between; this latticework is called *trabeculae*. Red bone marrow fills the spaces and is the site of hemopoeisis.

Cells that form bone tissue are called **osteoblasts**; when they become fixed in the dense bone matrix, they stop dividing but continue to maintain bone tissue as *osteocytes*. **Osteoclasts** break down the bone tissue. Remodeling is the continuous process of old bone being broken down by osteoclasts and replaced with stronger bone by osteoblasts.

Individual bones are classified by shape. The classifications include long bones, short bones, flat bones, irregular bones, and sesamoid bones. A typical long bone has an *epiphysis* at each end, which is the site of bone growth in length. Epiphyses are composed mainly of spongy bone covered by compact. The shaft of a long bone is the *diaphysis*. It is composed mainly of compact bone surrounding a hollow center called the *medullary cavity*. The medullary cavity is filled with yellow marrow or fat.

The **axial skeleton** (Fig. 7.4) consists of the skull, vertebral column, 12 pairs of ribs, and sternum. When including the 6 paired bones (ossicles) of the ear, the skull comprises 28 bones—14 facial bones and 14 cranial vault bones. The facial bones include two nasal bones, two maxillary bones, two zygomatic bones, one mandible (the only moveable bone of the skull), two palatine bones, one vomer, two lacrimal bones, and two inferior nasal conchae. The bones of the cranium are single occipital, frontal, ethmoid, and sphenoid bones, and the paired parietal and temporal bones. The ossicles of the ear (malleus, incus, and stapes) are part of the skull.

The vertebral column is divided into five subsections, as depicted in Figure 7.5. There are 7 cervical vertebrae, 12 thoracic vertebrae, 5 lumbar vertebrae, 5 sacral vertebrae (which fuse to form the sacrum), and the fused coccygeal vertebrae (known as the tailbone).

The **appendicular skeleton** (see Fig. 7.4) includes the shoulder and hip girdles, and the extremities. The upper portion consists of the pectoral or shoulder girdle formed by the clavicle and scapula, and the upper extremity. The bones of the arm are the humerus, radius and ulna, carpals (wrist bones), metacarpals (bones of the hand), and phalanges (bones of the fingers). The lower portion of the appendicular skeleton is made up of the pelvic girdle or os coxae. Each of the os coxae consists of a fused ilium, ischium, and pubis. Bones of the lower extremity include the femur (thigh bone), tibia and fibula, tarsals (ankle bones), metatarsals (bones of the foot), and phalanges (bones of the toes).

HESI Hint

Construct flash cards for learning the names, locations, and other features of bones and bone markings. Use mnemonic devices to recall the names and positions of bones, foramina, and other anatomic groups within the skeleton. Time and practice have proven to be successful learning strategies through the use of repetition.

Muscular System

Muscles produce movement by contracting in response to nervous stimulation. Each muscle cell, or muscle fiber, consists of myofibrils divided into segments called **sarcomeres**. Sarcomeres contain the myofilaments *actin*, a thin protein, and *myosin*, a thick protein. Muscle contraction occurs through the **sliding filament model**, in which the myosin binds to the actin, and pulls it toward the center of the sarcomere.

The skeletal muscles, which make up the muscular system, are also called voluntary muscles because they are under conscious control. Skeletal muscles must work in pairs: the muscle that performs a given movement is the *agonist* or *prime mover*, whereas the muscle that produces the opposite movement is the *antagonist*. Other muscles known as *synergists* may work in cooperation with the prime mover.

Muscles can be classified according to the movements they cause. For example, flexors reduce the angle at a joint, whereas extensors increase the angle. Abductors draw a limb away from the midline, and adductors return the limb back toward the body (Fig. 7.6).

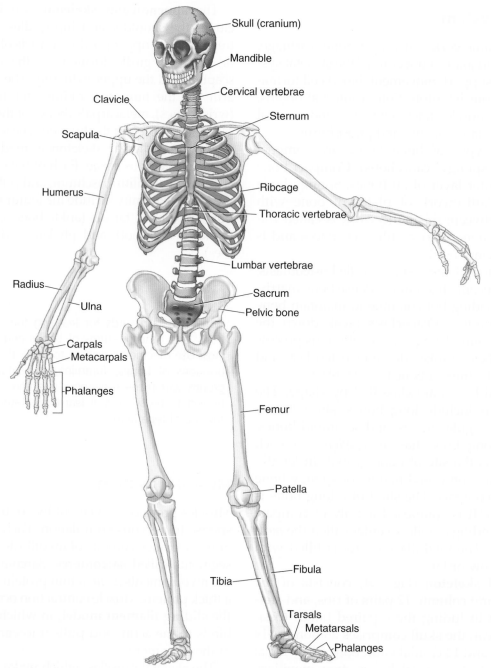

FIGURE 7.4 Bones colored beige are bones of the appendicular skeleton; bones colored green are bones of the axial skeleton. (From Muscolino: *Kinesiology: the skeletal system and muscle function,* ed 2, St Louis, 2011, Mosby.)

HESI Hint

The names of muscles are usually descriptive of their shape, location, and/or points of attachment. For example, deltoid is so named because "delta" refers to the capital Greek delta, which is triangular in shape. Occipitalis is located on the occipital bone. Sternocleidomastoid's attachments are the sternum, clavicle, and mastoid process of the skull.

Nervous System

The nervous system consists of the brain, the spinal cord, and the nerves (Figure 7.7). The central nervous system (CNS) comprises the spinal cord and brain, whereas the peripheral nervous system (PNS) is composed of all other nerves in the body, namely cranial nerves and peripheral

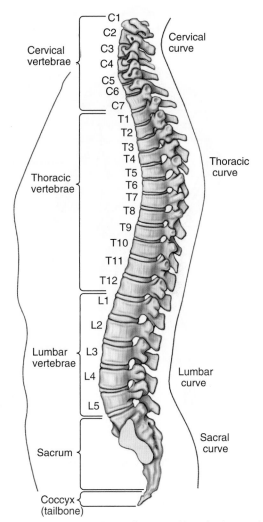

FIGURE 7.5 Vertebral column. (From Herlihy: *The human body in health and illness*, ed 5, St Louis, 2014, Saunders.)

nerves. The PNS is further divided into the somatic nervous system, which involves the skin, muscles, bones, and joints, and the **autonomic nervous system**, which controls functions such as digestion, heart rate, blood pressure, and urination. The two divisions of the autonomic nervous system are the *parasympathetic division* ("rest and digest") and the *sympathetic division* ("fight or flight").

The nervous system enables perception (seeing, hearing, tasting, smelling, and touching) of many of the changes that take place in the external and internal environments, and response to those changes. The nervous system is responsible for thinking, reasoning, remembering, and carrying out other abstract activities. It initiates body movements by skeletal muscles by supplying them with nerve impulses that cause contraction. It works closely with the endocrine glands,

correlating and integrating body functions such as digestion and reproduction.

All actions of the nervous system depend on the transmission of nerve impulses over **neurons**, or nerve cells, the functional units of the nervous system. The main parts of a neuron are the cell body, axon, and dendrites. Dendrites transmit the impulse toward the cell body, and axons transmit the impulse away from the cell body. Sensory (afferent) neurons transmit nerve impulses toward the CNS. Motor (efferent) neurons transmit nerve impulses away from the CNS toward the effector organs such as muscles, glands, and digestive organs.

The four major parts of the brain are the **cerebrum** (associated with sensory interpretation, movement, thinking, and personality), the **cerebellum** (responsible for muscular coordination), the **diencephalon** (contains the thalamus, which routes incoming sensory information to the appropriate part of the cerebrum, and the hypothalamus, which monitors many of the conditions of the body, controls the autonomic nervous system, and interacts with the endocrine system), and the **brainstem** (controls many vital functions such as respiration and heart rate).

The spinal cord is within the vertebral columns and is approximately 18 inches long and extends from the brainstem to the first or second lumbar vertebra (L1 or L2). Thirty-one pairs of spinal nerves exit the spinal cord. A *reflex* is a quick, automatic response to a stimulus. Simple spinal reflexes are those in which nerve impulses travel through the spinal cord only and do not reach the brain.

HESI Hint

Most reflex pathways involve impulses traveling to and from the brain in ascending and descending tracts of the spinal cord. Sensory impulses enter the posterior spinal cord, and motor impulses leave through the anterior spinal cord.

Endocrine System

The nervous and endocrine systems coordinate and control the body, but the endocrine system has more long-lasting and widespread effects. It also plays important roles in growth and sexual maturation. These two systems meet at the hypothalamus and pituitary gland. The hypothalamus governs the pituitary and is in turn controlled

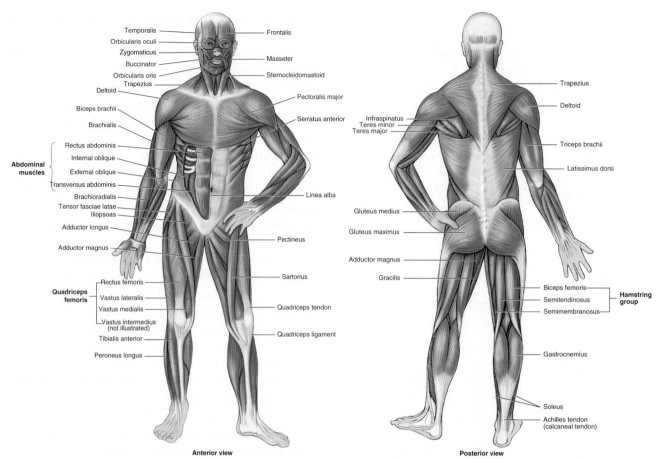

FIGURE 7.6 General overview of the body's musculature (anterior and posterior view). (From Herlihy: *The human body in health and illness,* ed 5, St Louis, 2014, Saunders.)

by the feedback of hormones in the blood as well as other conditions in the body. The endocrine glands, although widely distributed, are grouped together as a system because the main function of each gland is the production of hormones. Figure 7.8 shows the locations of the endocrine glands. Other organs, such as the stomach, small intestine, and kidneys, produce hormones as well.

Hormones are chemical messengers that control the growth, differentiation, and metabolism of specific target cells. There are two major groups of hormones, steroid and nonsteroid hormones. Steroid hormones enter the target cells and have a direct effect on the DNA of the nucleus. Nonsteroid hormones remain at the cell surface and act through a second messenger, usually a substance called *adenosine monophosphate,* AMP. Most hormones affect cell activity by altering the rate of protein synthesis.

HESI Hint

Multiple hormones are released during stress from the adrenal cortex, the hypothalamus, and the anterior and posterior pituitary gland. Cortisol, released from the adrenal cortex, is sometimes called the "stress hormone" because it reduces inflammation, raises the blood sugar level, and inhibits the release of histamine during long-term stress.

The pituitary gland is attached to the hypothalamus by a stalk called the *infundibulum.* The pituitary gland has two major portions: the anterior lobe (adenohypophysis) and the posterior lobe (neurohypophysis). Hormones of the adenohypophysis are called *tropic hormones* because they act mainly on other endocrine glands. They include:

• Somatotropin hormone (STH) or growth hormone (GH) – stimulates growth in all organs.

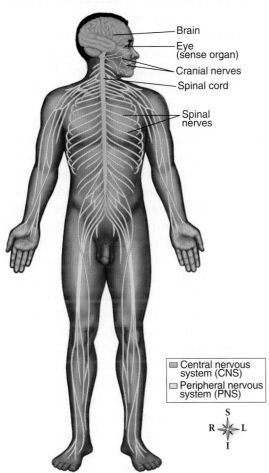

FIGURE 7.7 Major anatomical features of the nervous system include the brain, the spinal cord, and the individual nerves. The central nervous system (CNS) consists of the brain and spinal cord. The peripheral nervous system (PNS) includes all of the nerves and their branches. (From Patton KT, Thibodeau GA: *Anatomy and physiology*, ed 9, St Louis, 2016, Mosby.)

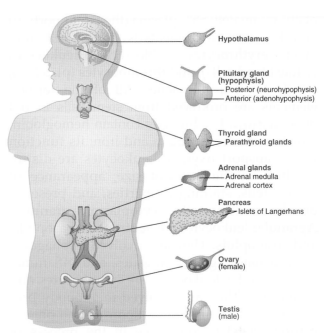

FIGURE 7.8 Locations of the endocrine glands. (From Kee: *Pharmacology: a patient-centered nursing process approach,* ed 8, St Louis, 2015, Saunders.)

- Adrenocorticotropic hormone (ACTH) – stimulates secretion of adrenal cortex hormones.
- Thyroid-stimulating hormone (TSH) – stimulates secretion of thyroid hormones.
- Follicle-stimulating hormone (FSH) – stimulates secretion of ovarian follicles and secretion of estrogens in females; stimulates sperm production in males.
- Luteinizing hormone (LH) – triggers ovulation in females; stimulates secretion of testosterone in males.
Hormones released from the posterior lobe of the pituitary include:
- Oxytocin – stimulates uterine contractions during labor; stimulates milk ejection from the mammary glands; it is also known as the bonding hormone.
- Antidiuretic hormone (ADH) – stimulates retention of water by the kidneys.
Other important endocrine glands include:
- Thyroid gland – secretes thyroid hormones which regulate metabolism, and calcitonin which decreases blood calcium levels.
- Parathyroid glands – secrete parathyroid hormone, which increases blood calcium levels.
- Adrenal glands – cortex secretes cortisol (discussed in the HESI Hint); medulla secretes adrenaline, which intensifies the sympathetic response.
- Pancreas – secretes insulin, which decreases blood glucose levels, and glucagon, which increases blood glucose levels.
- Gonads – ovaries secrete estrogens, which develop and maintain female sexual characteristics and progesterone, which maintains pregnancy; testes secrete testosterone, which develops and maintains male sexual characteristics.

Cardiovascular System

Blood transports oxygen, nutrients, enzymes, and hormones to body cells and carries away carbon dioxide and metabolic wastes. Whole blood consists of approximately 55% plasma (the liquid portion) and 45% formed elements (cells and cell fragments): **erythrocytes** (red blood cells), **leukocytes** (white blood cells), and **thrombocytes** (platelets), which are cell fragments. All of the formed elements are produced from stem cells in red bone marrow. Erythrocytes contain hemoglobin, which is made of protein and iron; its function is to transport oxygen. Leukocytes are distinguished on the basis of size, appearance of the nucleus, staining properties, and presence or absence of visible cytoplasmic granules. Agranular leukocytes are neutrophils, basophils, and eosinophils. They are involved in phagocytosis, defense against parasites, and inflammation. Granular leukocytes are lymphocytes and monocytes. They are involved in antibody production, cellular immune responses, and phagocytosis. Platelets are active in the process of blood clotting.

The heart is a double pump that sends blood to the lungs for oxygenation through the pulmonary circuit, and to the remainder of the body through the systemic circuit. Deoxygenated blood returning from the body is received by the right atrium, which sends it to the right ventricle. The right ventricle pumps this blood into the pulmonary arteries, which travel to the lungs. The blood becomes oxygenated in the lungs and returns to the left atrium of the heart. The oxygenated blood then enters the left ventricle, which pumps it into the aorta to be transported throughout the body.

Heart valves regulate blood flow. The tricuspid valve is between the right atrium and right ventricle; the bicuspid or mitral valve is between the left atrium and left ventricle. The pulmonary semilunar valve is between the right ventricle and pulmonary trunk (which splits into the pulmonary arteries). The aortic semilunar valve is between the left ventricle and the aorta.

Blood is supplied to the heart muscle (the myocardium) by the coronary arteries. Blood drains from the myocardium directly into the right atrium through the coronary sinus.

The heart has an intrinsic beat initiated by the sinoatrial node and transmitted along the conduction system through the myocardium. This wave of electrical activity is measured on an electrocardiogram (ECG). The cardiac cycle is the period from the end of one ventricular contraction to the end of the next ventricular contraction.

The contraction phase of the cycles is called systole; the relaxation phase is called diastole.

The vascular system includes arteries that carry oxygenated blood away from the heart, veins that carry deoxygenated blood toward the heart, and the capillaries. The capillaries, the smallest of vessels, are the sites of exchange of water, nutrients, and waste products between the blood and surrounding tissues. The systemic arteries begin with the aorta, which sends branches to all parts of the body. As arteries get farther away from the heart, they become thinner and thinner. The smallest arteries are called arterioles. Small veins called venules drain blood from the capillaries and send it to the veins. The veins parallel the arteries and most have the same names. The superior and inferior venae cava are the large veins that empty into the right atrium of the heart.

The walls of the arteries are thick and elastic, and they carry blood under high pressure. Vasoconstriction and vasodilation result from contraction and relaxation of smooth muscle in the arterial walls. These changes influence blood pressure and blood distribution to the tissues. The walls of the veins are thinner and less elastic than those of the arteries, and they carry blood under lower pressure. Figure 7.9 provides an overall view of the cardiovascular system.

HESI Hint

Deflections of the ECG do not represent the actual systole and diastole of the heart chambers. Instead, they represent the electrical activity that precedes the contraction-relaxation events of the myocardium. An analogy for this is the situation at a track meet when the starter's gun is fired before the runners start to run. The sound initiates the action. In the heart, the action potential is similar to firing the gun. The contraction starts just after the action potential passes over the muscle cells.

Respiratory System

Components of the respiratory system include the nose, pharynx, larynx, trachea, bronchi, lungs with their alveoli, diaphragm, and muscles surrounding the ribs. The structural plan of the respiratory system is shown in Figure 7.10. Respiration is controlled by the respiratory control center in the brainstem.

The respiratory system supplies oxygen to the body and eliminates carbon dioxide. **External**

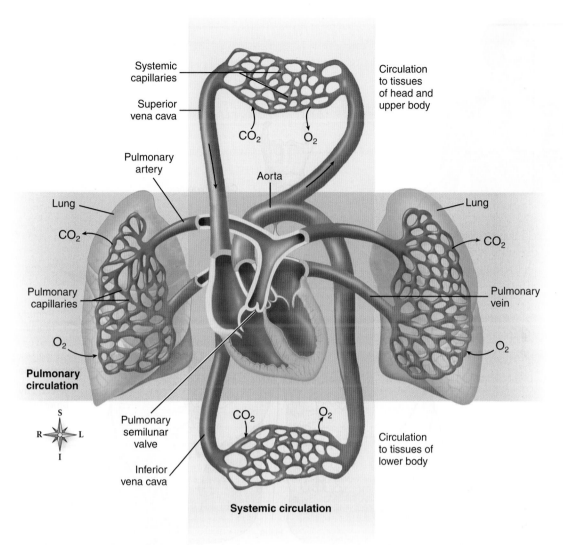

Systemic capillaries

Superior vena cava

Pulmonary artery

Aorta

Circulation to tissues of head and upper body

CO_2 O_2

Lung

Lung

CO_2

CO_2

Pulmonary capillaries

Pulmonary vein

O_2

O_2

Pulmonary circulation

S
R — L
I

Pulmonary semilunar valve

Inferior vena cava

CO_2 O_2

Circulation to tissues of lower body

Systemic circulation

FIGURE 7.9 Principal arteries of the body. (From Patton KT, Thibodeau GA: *Structure & function of the body,* ed 15, St Louis, 2016, Elsevier.)

respiration refers to the exchange of gases between the atmosphere and the blood through the alveoli. **Internal respiration** refers to the exchange of gases between the blood and the body cells. The passageways from the nasal cavities down to the alveoli conduct gases to and from the lungs. The upper passageways also serve to warm, filter, and moisten incoming air through mucous membranes and the movement of cilia.

Inhalation requires the contraction of the diaphragm to enlarge the thoracic cavity and draw air into the lungs. Exhalation is a passive process during which the lungs recoil as the respiratory muscles relax and the thorax decreases in size.

Most of the oxygen carried in the blood is bound to hemoglobin in red blood cells. Oxygen is released from hemoglobin as the concentration of oxygen drops in the tissues. Some carbon dioxide is carried on hemoglobin cells but most is converted to bicarbonate ion in the blood. Because this reaction also releases hydrogen ions, carbon dioxide is a regulator of blood pH.

HESI Hint

Using the familiar example of an inverted tree, the trachea can be visualized as the trunk and the two primary bronchi and their many subdivisions as the branches. This structure is often referred to as the bronchial tree. The analogy of a bunch of grapes can then be used to explain the terminal components of the respiratory tract, which include the alveolar ducts, alveolar sacs, and alveoli.

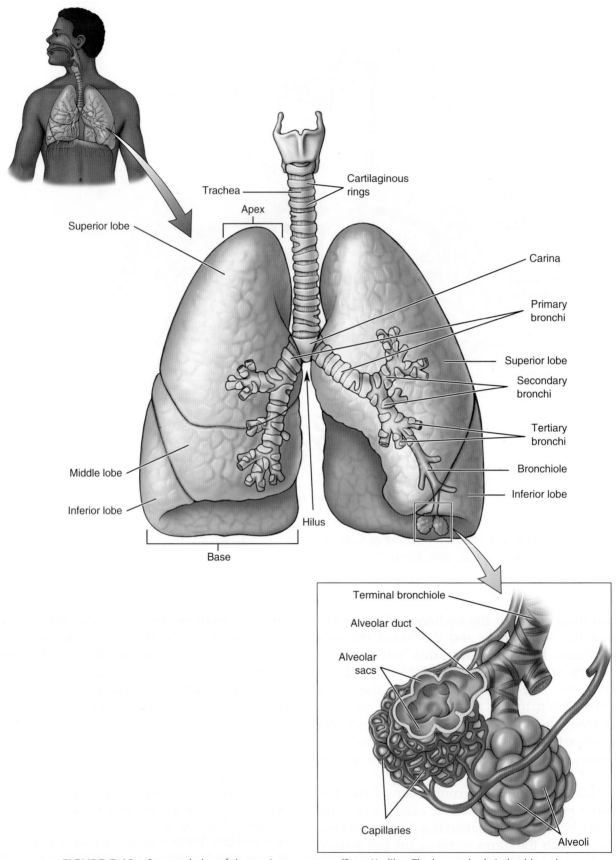

Trachea

Cartilaginous rings

Apex

Superior lobe

Carina

Primary bronchi

Superior lobe

Secondary bronchi

Tertiary bronchi

Bronchiole

Middle lobe

Inferior lobe

Inferior lobe

Hilus

Base

Terminal bronchiole

Alveolar duct

Alveolar sacs

Capillaries

Alveoli

FIGURE 7.10 Structural plan of the respiratory system. (From Herlihy: *The human body in health and illness,* ed 5, St Louis, 2014, Saunders.)

Digestive System

The digestive tract is a tube that consists of the mouth, pharynx, esophagus, stomach, small intestine, large intestine, rectum, and anus. The digestive tract has four main layers, from innermost to outer: the mucous membrane, the submucous layer, the muscular layer, and the serous layer. The accessory organs of digestion include the liver, pancreas, and gallbladder. The locations of the digestive organs are seen in Figure 7.11.

Food is ingested into the mouth where it is mechanically broken down by the teeth and tongue in the process of mastication (chewing). Saliva, produced by the three pairs of salivary glands, lubricates and dilutes the chewed food. Saliva contains an enzyme called amylase that starts the digestion of complex carbohydrates. A ball of food called a *bolus* is formed; swallowing forces it into the esophagus. The esophagus is a narrow tube leading from the pharynx to the stomach.

Food enters the stomach where gastric glands secrete hydrochloric acid that unwinds proteins so that the enzyme pepsin can digest them. The layers of muscle in the stomach wall churn and mix the bolus of food with gastric secretions, turning the mass into a soupy substance called *chyme*, which enters the small intestine.

The majority of digestion and absorption of food occur in the small intestine. The small intestine consists of three major regions: the duodenum, the jejunum, and the ileum. Bile, made by the liver and stored in the gallbladder, empties into the small intestine to emulsify fats. Secretions from the pancreas buffer the acidic chyme from the stomach, and contain enzymes such as lipase that digests fats, amylase that continues carbohydrate digestion, and protein-digesting enzymes. The small intestine also secretes digestive enzymes that finish digesting carbohydrates into monosaccharides, and protein-digesting enzymes.

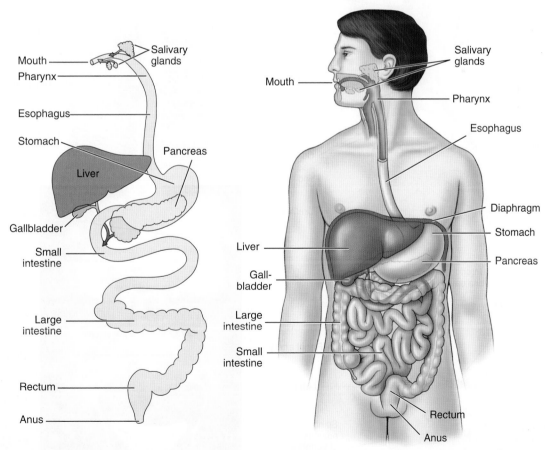

FIGURE 7.11 Location of the digestive organs. (From Herlihy: *The human body in health and illness,* ed 5, St Louis, 2014, Saunders.)

After digestion, nutrients are absorbed through the walls of the small intestine. Small finger-like projections called *villi* greatly increase the surface area of the intestinal wall. Amino acids and monosaccharides derived from proteins and carbohydrates are absorbed directly into the blood. Most of the fats are absorbed into the lymph *lacteals*; eventually, the fats are added to the bloodstream. The blood from the intestines enters the hepatic portal vein to be routed to the liver for decontamination, so nutrients can be processed before entering the systemic circulation.

The large intestine reabsorbs water and stores and eliminates undigested food. Here also are abundant bacteria, the intestinal flora. The large intestine is arranged into five portions: the ascending colon, the transverse colon, the descending colon, the sigmoid colon, and the rectum. The opening for defecation (expelling of feces) is the anus.

HESI Hint

During mastication, the teeth reduce ingested food material to smaller particles to increase surface area for chemical digestion. The muscular movements of the stomach and intestines also result in mechanical breakdown of food, thus increasing surface area for digestion.

Urinary System

The urinary system consists of two kidneys, two ureters, a urinary bladder, and the urethra. The kidneys filter the blood. The ureters are tubes that transport urine to the urinary bladder where urine is stored before urination through the urethra to the outside. Locations of urinary system organs are illustrated in Figure 7.12.

The functional units of the kidney are the **nephrons**. These small coiled tubes filter wastes out of the blood brought to the kidney by the

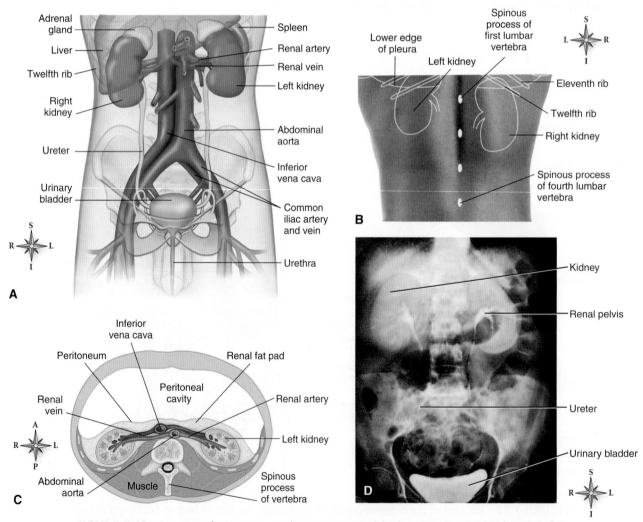

FIGURE 7.12 Location of urinary organs. (From Patton KT, Thibodeau GA: *Structure & function of the body*, ed 15, St Louis, 2016, Elsevier.)

renal artery. The actual filtration process occurs under the force of blood pressure through the glomerulus in Bowman's capsule of the nephron. As the glomerular filtrate passes through the nephron, components needed by the body, such as water, glucose, and ions, leave the nephron by diffusion and reenter the blood. Water is reabsorbed at the tubules of the nephron. The final product produced by the millions of nephrons per kidney is urine.

HESI Hint

The analogy of a wastewater treatment facility linked to an incredibly efficient recycling center may help explain the big picture of urinary system function. The central role of the kidneys is to serve as regulators of the internal environment. Most chemical exchanges with blood occur in the kidneys where they filter and process the blood to produce urine. In effect, they filter the body fluids of liquid sewage and at the same time retain essential chemicals and nutrients.

Reproductive System

The male and female sex organs (the testes and ovaries) produce gametes (sex cells) through meiosis and also produce hormones. These activities are under the control of tropic hormones from the pituitary gland. Reproductive activity is cyclic in women but continuous in men. Figures 7.13 and 7.14 show the location of male and female reproductive organs.

Male Reproductive System

In males, spermatozoa develop within the seminiferous tubules of each testis. The interstitial cells between the seminiferous tubules produce testosterone. This male hormone influences sperm cell development and also produces the male secondary sex characteristics such as increased facial hair and body hair as well as voice deepening. Once produced, the sperm are matured and stored in the epididymis of each testis. During ejaculation, the pathway for the sperm includes the vas deferens, ejaculatory duct, and urethra. Along the pathway are glands that produce the transport medium or semen. These include the seminal vesicles, prostate gland, and bulbourethral (Cowper's) glands.

Testicular activity is under the control of two anterior pituitary hormones. FSH regulates sperm production. Luteinizing hormone LH stimulates the interstitial cells to produce testosterone.

Female Reproductive System

In females, each month, under the influence of FSH, several eggs ripen within the ovarian follicles in the ovary. Estrogen produced by the

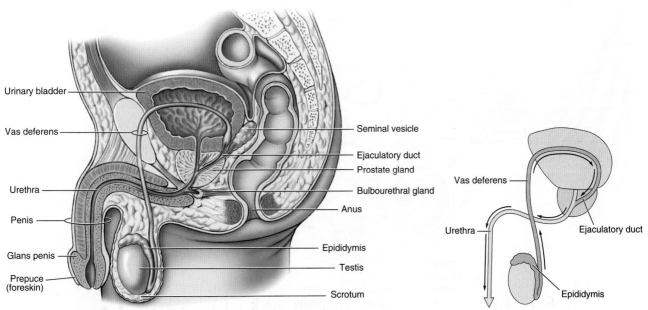

FIGURE 7.13 Male reproductive organs. (From Herlihy: *The human body in health and illness,* ed 5, St Louis, 2014, Saunders.)

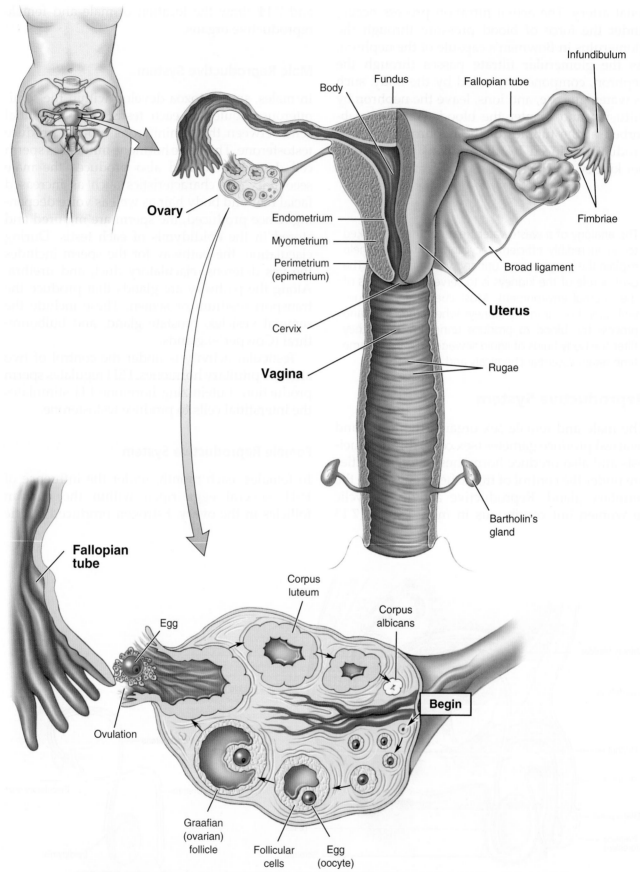

FIGURE 7.14 Female reproductive organs. (From Herlihy: *The human body in health and illness,* ed 5, St Louis, 2014, Saunders.)

follicle initiates the preparation of the endometrium of the uterus for pregnancy. At approximately day 14 of the cycle, a surge of LH is released from the pituitary gland, which stimulates ovulation and the conversion of the follicle to the corpus luteum. The corpus luteum secretes the hormones progesterone and estrogen, which further stimulate development of the endometrium. After ovulation, the egg is swept into the oviduct or fallopian tube. Fertilization, should it occur, happens while the egg is in the oviduct.

If fertilization occurs, the corpus luteum remains functional. If fertilization does not occur, the corpus luteum degenerates and menstruation begins. The fertilized egg or zygote travels to the uterus and implants itself within the endometrium. In the uterus, the developing embryo is nourished by the placenta, which is formed by maternal and embryonic tissues. During pregnancy, hormones from the placenta maintain the endometrium and prepare the mammary glands for breast milk production.

HESI Hint

To understand the processes involved in the menstrual cycle, first learn the functions of each hormone. Then focus on the specific actions of the hormones while moving through the cycle.

REVIEW QUESTIONS

1. Which statement is correct?
   A. Knee is distal to the ankle.
   B. Heart is inferior to the diaphragm.
   C. Hip is proximal to the knee.
   D. Wrist is proximal to the elbow.
2. Which plane separates the abdominal cavity from the thoracic cavity?
   A. Sagittal
   B. Transverse
   C. Frontal
   D. Coronal
3. A sample of tissue that has pillar-shaped cells arranged tightly together describes which type of epithelium?
   A. Squamous
   B. Cuboidal
   C. Columnar
   D. Transitional
4. How is the epidermis classified?
   A. Cell
   B. Tissue
   C. Organ
   D. System
5. Which type of tissue provides support and structure for the organs?
   A. Epithelial
   B. Connective
   C. Muscle
   D. Nervous
6. Within which epidermal layer of the skin does mitosis occur?
   A. Stratum lucidum
   B. Stratum granulosum
   C. Stratum corneum
   D. Stratum germinativum

7. The orthopedic surgeon informs the patient that the middle region of the humerus has been fractured. Which area is the surgeon describing?
   A. Epiphysis
   B. Articular cartilage
   C. Perichondrium
   D. Diaphysis
8. From superior to inferior, the sequence of the vertebral column is:
   A. Sacral, coccyx, thoracic, lumbar, and cervical
   B. Coccyx, sacral, lumbar, thoracic, and cervical
   C. Cervical, lumbar, thoracic, sacral, and coccyx
   D. Cervical, thoracic, lumbar, sacral, and coccyx
9. The cells that form bone are called:
   A. Osteoclasts
   B. Neuroglia
   C. Osteoblasts
   D. Neurons
10. Which statements are true about skeletal muscle? (Select all that apply.)
    A. The functional units are called nephrons.
    B. Synergists assist the prime mover in performing an action.
    C. Most of their actions are involuntary.
    D. Thin filaments slide over thick filaments during contraction.
11. Which chemicals are needed for a muscle cell to contract?
    A. Calcium and adenosine diphosphate (ADP)

B. Calcium and adenosine triphosphate (ATP)

C. Potassium and calcium

D. Sodium and calcium

12. Which term refers to the type of neuron an impulse travels from receptor to the spinal cord?
    A. Motor
    B. Sensory
    C. Tract
    D. Efferent

13. Which chemical does parathyroid hormone regulate?
    A. Magnesium
    B. Calcium
    C. Calcitonin
    D. Sodium

14. Which area of the brain controls vital functions such as respiration and heart rate?
    A. Diencephalon
    B. Cerebellum

C. Cerebrum

D. Brainstem

15. Bile is secreted into which organ?
    A. Small intestine
    B. Liver
    C. Large intestine
    D. Stomach

16. What is the role of progesterone in the female reproductive system?
    A. Stimulates ovulation
    B. Conversion of the follicle to the corpus luteum
    C. Development of the endometrium
    D. Stimulates the start of menstruation

ANSWERS TO REVIEW QUESTIONS

1. C
2. B
3. C
4. B
5. B
6. D
7. D
8. D

9. C
10. B, D
11. B
12. B
13. B
14. D
15. A
16. C

PHYSICS

Members of the health professions, particularly medical imaging professionals, use the fundamental principles of physics on a daily basis as they relate to various aspects of imaging science such as radiation safety, radiation dose limits, patient and health professional protection, and patient positioning. Safety and high-quality image production are the goals of all who work within the imaging sciences. Therefore, it is essential that students entering the health professions as medical imaging professionals understand the fundamental principles of physics.

The purpose of this chapter is to review the fundamentals of physics relevant to those considering medical imaging careers. In particular, it is a review of the behavior of matter under various conditions and an understanding of basic phenomena in our natural world. Mastery of these basic principles of physics is an integral step toward a career as a health professional in medical imaging.

CHAPTER OUTLINE

Nature of Motion	Uniform Circular Motion	Light
Projectile Motion	Kinetic Energy and Potential Energy	Optics
Newton's Laws of Motion	Linear Momentum and Impulse	Atomic Structure
Friction	Universal Gravitation	The Nature of Electricity
Rotation	Waves and Sound	Magnetism and Electricity

KEY TERMS

Acceleration	Joules	Reflection
Average Speed	Kinetic Energy	Refraction
Binding Energy	Law of Universal Gravitation	Scalar Quantity
Centripetal Acceleration	Momentum	Valence Electrons
Force	Newton	Vector Quantity
Friction	Potential Energy	Velocity
Impulse Equation	Projectile Motion	

Nature of Motion

Speed and Velocity

A study of the behavior of matter begins with an understanding of the nature of motion. The most fundamental concept to comprehend is average speed. **Average speed** is defined as the distance an object travels divided by the time the object travels without regard to direction of travel. This concept is represented mathematically by the following equation, where v_{av} = average speed, d = distance, and t = time:

$$\text{Average speed } (v_{av}) = \frac{\text{Distance}}{\text{Time}} = \frac{d}{t}$$

SAMPLE PROBLEM

1. A car travels 3,200 m in 20 min. What is the average speed of the car?
   A. 2.67 m/s
   B. 267 m/s
   C. 8.8 m/s
   D. 88 m/s

Answer

A—Average speed is the distance an object travels divided by the time the object travels. First, the answers must be expressed in m/s; therefore, the time of travel by the car must be converted from minutes to seconds before the average speed is determined:

$$\frac{X}{20 \text{ min}} = \frac{60 \text{ s}}{1 \text{ min}}$$

$$X = \frac{60 \text{ s} \times 20 \text{ min}}{1 \text{ min}}$$

$$x = 1200 \text{ s}$$

Dividing the distance traveled by the car (3,200 m) by the new value for time traveled by the car (1200 seconds) determines that the average speed of the car is 2.67 m/s.

$$\text{Average speed } (v_{av}) = \frac{\text{Distance}}{\text{time}}$$

$$\text{Average speed} = \frac{3,200 \text{ m}}{1,200 \text{ s}}$$

$$\text{Average speed} = 2.67 \text{ m/s}$$

Velocity

An important related concept is velocity. **Velocity** refers to speed in a specific direction. Speed is a **scalar quantity** (quantity described simply by a numeric value) and is expressed in units of magnitude. Velocity is a **vector quantity** (quantity describing the time rate of change of an object's position) and must be expressed in both units of magnitude (i.e., speed) and direction of motion.

The average velocity of an object is determined by averaging the initial speed and the final speed of the object (add the two together and divide by 2). This concept is represented mathematically by the following equation, where v_f = final velocity and v_i = initial velocity.

$$v_{av} = \frac{v_f + v_i}{2}$$

Often, objects in motion change velocity over a period of time. Such a change in motion is called **acceleration** and is defined as the rate of change in velocity over a period of time. Acceleration is a vector quantity and is expressed in terms of magnitude and direction. This concept is represented mathematically by the following equation, where a = acceleration, v_f = final velocity, v_i = initial velocity, and Δt = the change in time.

$$\text{Acceleration } (a) = \frac{\Delta \text{Velocity}}{\Delta \text{Time}} = \frac{\Delta v}{\Delta t} = \frac{v_f - v_i}{\Delta t}$$

SAMPLE PROBLEM

2. A wagon is set in motion. The wagon has an initial speed of 20 m/s and moves for 35 seconds. At the end of 35 seconds, the wagon's speed is 50 m/s. What is the magnitude of the wagon's acceleration?
   A. 0.3 m/s²
   B. 0.86 m/s²
   C. 1.37 m/s²
   D. 2.4 m/s²

Answer

B—Acceleration is determined by dividing the change in the wagon's velocity (final velocity [50 m/s] – initial velocity [20 m/s] = 30 m/s) by the length of time the wagon was in motion

(35 seconds), indicating the wagon is accelerating at 0.86 m/s².

$$\text{Acceleration } (a) = \frac{v_f - v_i}{\Delta t}$$

$$a = \frac{50\,\text{m/s} - 20\,\text{m/s}}{35\,\text{s}}$$

$$a = \frac{30\,\text{m/s}}{35\,\text{s}}$$

$$A = 0.86\,\text{m/s}^2$$

Projectile Motion

The acceleration of objects released above the surface of the earth is influenced by the force of gravity. Gravity, assuming no wind resistance, accelerates an object released above the earth's surface at a rate of 9.8 m/s². For example, if a rock is released from rest and falls toward the earth, the speed of the rock will increase by 9.8 m/s for every second the object falls. At the end of 3 s, the object will have a speed of 29.4 m/s and a velocity of 29.4 m/s in the direction toward earth's surface.

It is also possible for an object to display two types of motion simultaneously. This motion is generally called **projectile motion**. If a can is kicked from the edge of a cliff, the can will move horizontally at the same time it falls toward earth (Fig. 8.1). The horizontal motion is not an accelerated motion; therefore, horizontal distance (d_x) is a function of velocity (v_x) and time (*t*) based on the following mathematic expression, where the *x* subscript is used to denote motion along the horizontal plane (x axis).

$$d_x = v_x t$$

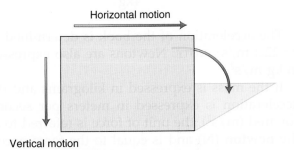

Horizontal motion

Vertical motion

FIGURE 8.1   Projectile motion.

The vertical motion is more complicated. Gravity is acting vertically, so the velocity along the vertical plane (y axis) is constantly changing. The following mathematic expressions represent several methods of describing vertical motion, where v_f = final velocity, v_i = initial velocity, *a* = acceleration, *d* = distance, and *t* = time.

$$v_f^2 = v_i^2 + 2ad$$

$$d = \frac{1}{2}at^2 + v_i t$$

$$v_f = v_i + at$$

3. A ball is kicked off a cliff that is 23.7 m tall. The horizontal speed given to the ball is 14.0 m/s. Assuming there is no air resistance, how far out from the base of the cliff will the ball land?
   A. 14.0 m
   B. 47.4m
   C. 4.84 m
   D. 30.8 m

Answer

D—The problem provides values for the vertical distance (height of cliff), vertical acceleration (gravitational constant), and initial vertical velocity (at rest on cliff, thus 0). The first step is to calculate time of flight. The following equation can be transformed to determine the time of flight.

$$d = \frac{1}{2}at^2 + v_i t$$

$v_i t$ drops out of the equation because the initial vertical velocity is 0.

$$d = \frac{1}{2}at^2$$

Convert the equation to solve for time.

$$t = \sqrt{\frac{d^*2}{a}}$$

$$t = \sqrt{\frac{23.7^*2}{9.8}}$$

$$t = 2.2\,\text{s}$$

Once the time of flight is determined, insert the appropriate values into the horizontal distance equation to solve for horizontal distance.

$$d_x = v_x t$$
$$d_x = 14.0 \text{ m/s} \times 2.2 \text{ s}$$
$$d_x = 30.8 \text{ m}$$

Assuming no air resistance, the ball will land 30.8 m from the cliff.

Newton's Laws of Motion

Force

Before delving into Newton's laws of motion, a brief discussion of force is necessary. **Force** is defined as a push or pull on an object. When two forces are equal in magnitude and in opposing directions, they cancel each other out and result in a balanced force. However, if one of the two forces is greater than the other, an unbalanced force exists and with it acceleration. Net force is simply the sum of the individual forces acting on an object. Keep in mind that the + and − signs are used to indicate direction of force and the mathematic rules associated with summing negative and positive numbers apply.

Newton's First Law of Motion

Newton's first law of motion states that a body at rest will remain at rest, and a body in motion will remain in motion with a constant velocity, unless acted on by an unbalanced force (a force not opposed by one of equal magnitude and in the opposite direction). Newton's second law of motion states that an unbalanced force will cause acceleration, and this acceleration is directly proportional to the unbalanced force. This relationship is expressed mathematically as follows, where F = force, a = acceleration, and k = the constant of proportionality.

$$F = ka$$

Newton's Second Law of Motion

When used in Newton's second law of motion, the constant of proportionality (k) is equal to the mass of the object. Therefore, Newton's second law is expressed mathematically as follows, where F = force, m = mass, and a = acceleration.

$$F = ma$$

SAMPLE PROBLEM

4. A book rests on a tabletop. The book has a mass of 4 kg and is acted on by two forces. The force pushing to the right is 56 N, whereas the force pushing to the left is 145 N. Determine the magnitude of the acceleration of the book, assuming there is no friction between the book and the table.
   A. 12.5 m/s²
   B. 22.3 m/s²
   C. 37.4 m/s²
   D. 43.7 m/s²

Answer

B—To determine the acceleration of the book, it is necessary to first determine the net force acting on the book. Remember that the net force acting on the book is simply the sum of all forces acting on the book. Because the two forces are opposing each other, one force is considered a positive force and the other a negative force. Therefore, net force is represented by the following mathematic equation and is determined to be 89 N to the left.

$$\text{NetForce} = F_{left} + (-) F_{right}$$
$$\text{NetForce} = 145 \text{ N} + (-) 56 \text{ N}$$
$$\text{NetForce} = 89 \text{ N} \leftarrow$$

Once the net force is determined, use Newton's second law equation to determine the magnitude of acceleration of the book.

$$F = ma$$

First, convert the formula to solve for acceleration.

$$a = \frac{F}{m}$$
$$a = \frac{89N}{4kg}$$

The acceleration of the book is determined to be 22.3 m/s². NOTE: Newtons are also expressed in kg-m/s².

If the mass is expressed in kilograms and the acceleration is expressed in meters per second squared (m/s²), the unit of force is referred to as the **newton** (N) and is equal to the force necessary to accelerate a mass of one kilogram one meter per second per second. Weight is simply a specialized case of Newton's second law. Weight can be stated mathematically as follows, where m = mass in kilograms and g = 9.8 m/s² (i.e., the rate of acceleration associated with gravity).

$$W = mg$$

SAMPLE PROBLEM

5. An object has a mass of 3,100 g. Determine the weight of the object on earth.
   A. 30.38 N
   B. 303.8 N
   C. 3038 N
   D. 30380 N

Answer

A—To determine the weight of the object on earth, first convert the units of mass to kilograms (3,100 g = 3.1 kg). Second, insert the appropriate values into the weight equation.

$$W = mg$$
$$W = 3.1 \text{ kg} \times 9.8 \text{ m/s}^2$$
$$W = 30.38 \text{ N}$$

The weight of the object on earth is determined to be 30.38 N.

Newton's Third Law of Motion

Newton's third law of motion states that for every action there must be an equal and opposite reaction.

Friction

Friction is a force that opposes motion and is expressed in newtons. If a box (Fig. 8.2) is slid on a surface at a constant rate by an applied force, we can deduce that friction is present and is opposing

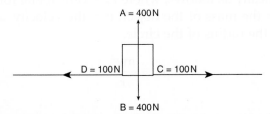

FIGURE 8.2 Depiction of a box being slid on a surface at a constant rate by an applied force.

the motion of the box. Because there is no acceleration of the box, it is clear that friction is present and all forces are balanced. This relationship of balanced forces is represented in the diagram. Note that the normal force (A) and the weight (B) are balanced. The applied force (C) is to the right and has a magnitude of 100 N. The frictional force (D) is to the left and must also be 100 N if the box has no acceleration.

SAMPLE PROBLEM

6. A box is pulled to the right by a rope attached to the box. The force applied to the rope is 470 N. As the box slides along the floor, there is a frictional force between the box and the floor that has a magnitude of 325 N. Determine the magnitude of the net force acting on the box.
   A. 795 N
   B. 470 N
   C. 325 N
   D. 145 N

Answer

D—To determine the magnitude of the net force acting on the box, remember that the magnitude of the net force acting on the box is simply the sum of all forces acting on the box. Because the two forces are opposing each other, applied force to the right and friction to the left, the magnitude of the net force is represented by the following mathematic equation and is determined to be 145 N to the right.

$$NetForce = F_{right} + (-)F_{left}$$
$$NetForce = 470 \text{ N} + (-)325 \text{ N}$$
$$NetForce = 145 \text{ N} \rightarrow$$

Rotation

In addition to displaying linear motion, an object may display a rotating or circular motion. The relationship between the angular displacement and the radius of the circle is expressed mathematically as follows, where θ = the angular displacement, S = arc length, and r = radius of the circle through which the object is moving.

$$\theta = \frac{S}{r}$$

Box 8.1 Mathematic Expressions Describing Linear and Rotational Motion

Linear Motion	Rotational Motion
$d = v_{av}t$	$\theta = \omega_{av}t$
$v_f = v_i + at$	$\omega_f = \omega_i + \alpha t$
$d = \dfrac{1}{2}at^2 + v_i t$	$\theta = \dfrac{1}{2}\alpha t^2 + \omega_i t$
$v_f^2 = v_i^2 + 2ad$	$\omega_f^2 = \omega_i^2 + 2\alpha\theta$

The average speed of the circular motion can be described by looking at the number of rotations or revolutions an object makes in a given time. The angular speed is the number of radians completed in a given time unit. This is expressed mathematically as follows, where ω = angular speed, θ = the angular displacement, and t = time. When the mathematic expression is considered, it is important to remember that there are 2π radians in one revolution.

$$\omega = \frac{\Delta\theta}{\Delta t}$$

It is also possible to have an angular acceleration as a spinning or rotating object gains or loses speed. This is expressed mathematically as follows, where α = angular acceleration, ω = angular speed, and t = time.

$$\alpha = \frac{\Delta\omega}{\Delta t}$$

The relationship between linear motion and rotational motion is analogous and conforms to Newton's laws. Box 8.1 provides a description of the relationship between the mathematic expressions describing linear motion and those describing rotational motion. Beside each linear motion formula is its rotational motion counterpart. The expressions have been defined and applied within this chapter.

SAMPLE PROBLEM

7. If a bicycle wheel goes from 57 revolutions/s to 93 revolutions/s in 15 s, what is the angular acceleration of the wheel?
   A. 0.45 revolutions/s²
   B. 1.36 revolutions/s²
   C. 2.4 revolutions/s²
   D. 3.73 revolutions/s²

Answer

C—To determine the angular acceleration, divide the change in angular speed by the time it took to complete the change in speed.

$$\omega_f = \omega_i + \alpha t$$

Convert the equation to solve for angular acceleration (*a*).

$$\alpha = \frac{\omega_f - \omega_i}{t}$$

$$\alpha = \frac{93\text{ rev/s} - 57\text{ rev/s}}{15\text{ s}}$$

$$\alpha = 2.4\text{ rev/s}^2$$

Uniform Circular Motion

It is possible for an object to experience acceleration even though the object is moving at a constant speed. This is possible because acceleration is a vector quantity and is defined as a change in velocity over a change in time. Velocity has a magnitude and a direction, so even though the speed or magnitude of the velocity is constant, the direction could be changing. In uniform circular motion, this is exactly what is happening. Therefore, the object is undergoing an acceleration called a **centripetal acceleration** (rotational motion equivalent of acceleration). Centripetal acceleration is represented mathematically as follows, where a_c = centripetal acceleration, v = the speed of the object in meters per second, and r = the radius of the circle.

$$a_c = \frac{v^2}{r}$$

Because there is a centripetal acceleration, there must also be a centripetal force. Newton's law states that force is a function of mass and acceleration; therefore, centripetal force must be a function of mass of an object and centripetal acceleration. This relationship is expressed mathematically as follows, where F_c = centripetal force, m = the mass of the object, v = the velocity, and r = the radius of the circle.

$$F_c = \frac{mv^2}{r}$$

The direction of both the force and the acceleration must be toward the center of the circle. Think of whirling a stone attached to a string in a horizontal circle. The tension in the cord keeps the stone moving in a circular path by pulling inward on the stone.

SAMPLE PROBLEM

8. A 0.25-kg rubber ball is spun in a circle on a 1.7-m string. If the string breaks at 20 N of tension, how fast must the rock be moving?
   A. 11.66 m/s
   B. 8.7 m/s
   C. 1.7 m/s
   D. 0.92 m/s

Answer

A—The centripetal force (20 N) is supplied by the tension in the string. The radius of the circle is 1.7 m, and the mass of the rubber ball is 0.25 kg. After these values are inserted in the centripetal force equation, the speed of the rubber ball is determined to be 11.66 m/s.

$$F_c = \frac{mv^2}{r}$$

Convert the equation to solve for velocity.

$$v = \sqrt{\frac{F_c r}{m}}$$

$$v = \sqrt{\frac{(20\,N)(1.7\,m)}{0.25\,kg}}$$

$$v = 11.66\,m/s$$

Kinetic Energy and Potential Energy

Kinetic energy of an object is the energy resulting from the motion of the object and is represented by the following equation, where KE = kinetic energy, m = mass of the object, and v = velocity.

$$KE = \frac{1}{2}mv^2$$

In this equation, mass must be expressed in kilograms and velocity must be expressed in meters per second.

The **potential energy** of an object is the energy the object has because of its position and is expressed by the following equation, where PE = potential energy, m = mass of the object, g = acceleration caused by gravity, and h = the height at which the object is located above the ground.

$$PE = mgh$$

In this equation, mass must be expressed in kilograms, gravity is a constant expressed as 9.8 m/s², and height is expressed in meters.

Kinetic energy and potential energy are scalar quantities and are expressed in units called **joules**. A joule is a newton-meter or a kilogram-meter squared per second squared (kg-m²/s²). Remember that the law of conservation of energy states that energy must be conserved; therefore, kinetic energy and potential energy can be interchanged if we assume that there is no friction or air resistance present.

SAMPLE PROBLEM

9. A car has a mass of 1,087 kg and is moving at 19 m/s. How much kinetic energy does the car have as a result of its motion?
   A. 20,653 J
   B. 10,326.5 J
   C. 392,407 J
   D. 196,203.5 J

Answer

D—The problem provides values for mass and velocity; after the appropriate values for kinetic energy are inserted into the equation, the kinetic energy as a result of the car's motion is determined to be 196,203.5 J.

$$KE = \frac{1}{2}mv^2$$

$$KE = \frac{1}{2}(1,087\,kg)(19\,m/s)^2$$

$$KE = 196,203.5\,J$$

Linear Momentum and Impulse

Considering Newton's second law of motion in the following slightly different form allows for the development of a new relationship.

$$F = \frac{m\Delta v}{\Delta t}$$

If both sides of this equation are multiplied by Δt, a new relationship between force and time is established and expressed as follows:

$$F\Delta t = m\Delta v$$

The new relationship is referred to as the **impulse equation** because a force applied over a period of time is an impulse. This impulse causes a change in velocity of the object, which results in a change in momentum of the object. **Momentum** is defined as the amount of motion displayed by an object and is represented by the following mathematical equation, where p = the momentum in kilogram-meters per second, m = the mass in kilograms, and Δv = the change in velocity of the object.

$$p = m\Delta v$$

Momentum is a vector quantity, which means we must have both magnitude and direction to completely express momentum. Momentum must always be conserved, so the momentum before an interaction must equal the momentum after an interaction. This relationship is expressed mathematically as follows, where m_1 and m_2 = masses 1 and 2, v_1' and v_2' = the initial velocities of objects 1 and 2, and v_1 and v_2 = the final velocities of objects 1 and 2 after the interaction.

$$m_1 v_1' + m_2 v_2' = m_1 v_1 + m_2 v_2$$

SAMPLE PROBLEM

10. A 600-g basketball traveling at 13.4 m/s strikes a motionless 875-g wood panel. If the basketball bounces off the wood panel at 8.7 m/s, how fast will the wood panel be moving?
   A. 0.045 m/s
   B. 0.89 m/s
   C. 1.57 m/s
   D. 3.22 m/s

Answer

D—With the conservation of momentum equation, with the basketball established as mass 1 and the wood panel established as mass 2, and with the initial velocity of the wood panel being 0, the speed of the wood panel after impact with the basketball is determined to be 3.22 m/s.

$$m_1 v_1 + m_2 v_2 = m_1 v_1' + m_2 v_2'$$

Convert the equation to solve for the speed of the block after impact (v_2').

$$v_2' = \frac{m_1 v_1 + m_2 v_2 = m_1 v_1'}{m_2}$$

$$v_2' = \frac{(600 \times 13.4 \text{ m/s}) = (875 \times 0) - (600 \times 8.7 \text{ m/s})}{875 \text{ g}}$$

$$v_2' = 3.22 \text{ m/s}$$

Universal Gravitation

Newton stated that every object in the universe attracts every other object in the universe. This statement is known as the **law of universal gravitation** and is expressed mathematically as follows, where F = force of attraction, m_1 and m_2 = the masses of objects 1 and 2 expressed in kilograms, G = the universal gravitation constant (6.67×10^{-11} Nm^2/kg^2), and r = the distance between the two objects expressed in meters.

$$F = \frac{Gm_1 m_2}{r^2}$$

SAMPLE PROBLEM

11. If object 1 of mass 372 kg is placed 834 m from object 2 of mass 860 kg, what force of attraction exists between the two objects?
   A. 1.24×10^{-7} N
   B. 2.48×10^{-7} N
   C. 4.14×10^{-10} N
   D. 9.25×10^{-11} N

Answer

D—When all values are correctly placed in the universal gravitation equation, the force of attraction between the two masses is determined to be 9.25×10^{-11} N.

$$F = \frac{Gm_1 m_2}{r^2}$$

$$F = \frac{\left(6.67 \times 10^{-11} \text{ Nm}^2/\text{kg}^2\right)(372 \text{ kg})(834 \text{ kg})}{473 \text{ m}}$$

$$F = (372 \text{ kg})(834 \text{ kg})$$

$$F = 9.25 \times 10^{-11}$$

Waves and Sound

To review waves, it is helpful to take a look at the vocabulary associated with waves in Box 8.2 and the illustration in Figure 8.3.

The frequency of the wave and the period of the wave are inversely related and expressed mathematically as follows, where f = the frequency and T = the period.

$$f = \frac{1}{T}$$

Box 8.2 Wave Vocabulary

Crest: High point of a wave.
Trough: Low point of a wave.
Amplitude: Maximum displacement from equilibrium.
Wavelength: Distance between successive identical parts of a wave.
Frequency: Vibrations or oscillations per unit of time (number of waves per unit time). Frequency is expressed in vibrations per second and is measured in hertz (s^{-1}).

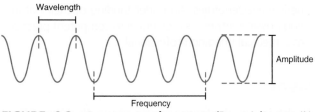

FIGURE 8.3 Components of a wave. (From Johnston JN, Fauber TL: *Essentials of radiographic physics and imaging,* ed 2, St Louis, 2016, Elsevier Mosby.)

and

$$T = \frac{1}{f}$$

Waves are produced by objects that vibrate or show simple harmonic motion. A wave is a disturbance or pulse that travels through a medium or space. Waves are carriers of energy that travel in the form of light, sound, microwaves, ultraviolet light, x-rays, gamma rays, television, and radio. There are two types of waves, mechanical and electromagnetic.

Mechanical Waves

Each type of mechanical wave is associated with some material or substance called the *medium* for that type. As the wave travels through the medium, the particles that make up the medium undergo displacements of various kinds, depending on the nature of the wave. Examples of these would be sound, water, and seismic.

Electromagnetic Waves

Electromagnetic waves do not require a medium for transmission. These waves are produced by electricity and magnetism and make up the electromagnetic spectrum. They are pure energy and travel as electric and magnetic disturbances in space (Fig. 8.4). All these waves travel at the speed of light (3×10^8 m/s). The components of the electromagnetic spectrum are radio waves,

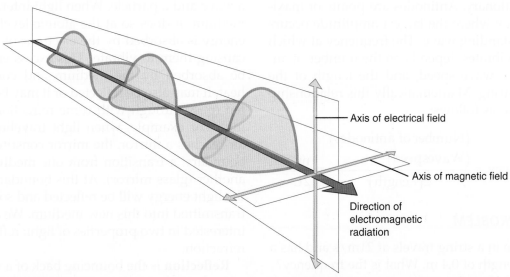

FIGURE 8.4 Electromagnetic radiation is an electric and magnetic disturbance in space. (From Johnston JN, Fauber TL: *Essentials of radiographic physics and imaging,* ed 2, St Louis, 2016, Elsevier Mosby.)

microwaves, infrared light, visible light, ultraviolet light, x-rays, and gamma rays.

Classification of Waves

Waves are classified by the way they displace matter or how they cause matter to vibrate. The wave is either transverse or longitudinal in nature. Transverse waves cause the particles of the medium to vibrate perpendicular to the direction the wave travels. Longitudinal or compressional waves cause the particles of the medium to vibrate parallel to the direction of the wave. With both longitudinal and transverse waves, the particles of the medium vibrate but *do not* travel with the wave. Longitudinal waves require a medium to be transmitted. The speed at which a wave travels through a medium is determined by the frequency and the wavelength of the wave. This relationship is expressed mathematically as follows, where f = frequency and λ = the wavelength.

$$\text{Speed} = f\lambda$$

The amplitude of a wave is proportional to the potential energy content of the wave. Therefore, the higher the wave, the greater the stored energy it is carrying. The higher the frequency, the more kinetic energy the wave possesses because speed $(v) = f\lambda$ and $KE = \frac{1}{2} mv^2$.

When a string is plucked, a wave will reflect back and forth from one end of the string to the other, creating nodes and antinodes. This is called a *standing wave* because it appears to stand still. Nodes are points along the standing wave that remain stationary. Antinodes are points of maximum energy where the largest amplitude occurs along the standing wave. The frequency at which the string vibrates depends on the number of antinodes, the wave speed, and the length of the vibrating string. Mathematically this relationship is expressed as follows:

$$\text{Frequency} = \frac{(\text{Number of antinodes})(\text{Wavespeed})}{2(\text{Length})} = \frac{nv}{2L}$$

SAMPLE PROBLEM

12. A wave in a string travels at 21m/s and has a wavelength of 0.4 m. What is the frequency?
    A. 0.02 Hz
    B. 8.4 Hz

C. 52.5 Hz
D. 67 Hz

Answer

C—To determine the frequency of a wave given the speed and wavelength, simply divide the speed of the wave by the wavelength. After insertion of the appropriate values in the following equation, the frequency of the wave is determined to be 52.5 Hz.

$$\text{speed} = f\lambda$$

Convert the equation to solve for frequency (f).

$$f = \frac{\text{speed}}{\lambda}$$

$$f = \frac{21 \text{ m/s}}{0.4 \text{ m}}$$

$$f = 52.5 \text{ Hz}$$

HESI Hint

Medical imaging, whether radiography, magnetic resonance imaging, or ultrasound, deals with electromagnetic waves/energies. An understanding of their nature and physical attributes is essential to competent practice as a medical imaging professional.

Light

Light is an electromagnetic wave that travels at 3.0×10^8 m/s. Light needs no medium through which to travel and is a result of electric and magnetic interactions. Light exhibits properties of both a wave and a particle. When light interacts with a medium, it does so at the atomic level. The light energy is absorbed by the electrons of the atoms, causing them to vibrate. This excess energy may be absorbed by the medium and converted to heat. It may also be reflected or it may be transmitted (pass through with some refraction or bending). For example, when light traveling through air reaches a mirror, the mirror constitutes a new boundary, a transition from one medium (air) to another (glass mirror). At this boundary, some of the light energy will be reflected and some will be transmitted into this new medium. We are mainly interested in two properties of light: reflection and refraction.

Reflection is the bouncing back of a wave from a barrier or from a boundary between two media, as depicted in Figure 8.5. There are a few terms

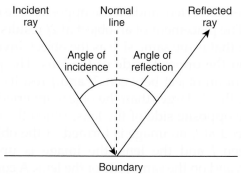

FIGURE 8.5 Reflection is a wave bouncing back from a barrier or from a boundary between two media.

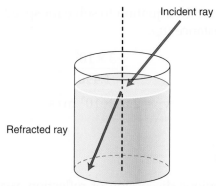

FIGURE 8.6 Light ray refracted in a container of water.

important to the discussion of reflection. Incident wave is the wave that strikes the barrier (or boundary). *Reflected wave* is the wave that bounces off and leaves the barrier. The *normal line* is a reference line that is drawn perpendicular to a barrier. The *angle of incidence* is the angle between the normal line and the incident wave. The *angle of reflection* is the angle between the normal line and the reflected wave. Applying the mirror example to Figure 8.5, the mirror would be the boundary, the incident ray would be the light traveling to the mirror, and the reflected ray would be the light traveling away from the mirror. The law of reflection states that when a wave disturbance is reflected at a boundary of a transmitting medium, the angle of incidence must equal the angle of reflection.

HESI Hint

X-rays and gamma rays also exhibit properties of both a wave and a particle referred to as *wave/particle duality.* Understanding this property aids in understanding how these radiant energies interact with matter.

Refraction is the bending of a wave as it passes at an angle from one medium into another if the speed of propagation differs. That is, refraction is caused by the change in speed of a wave as it transitions from one medium to the next. Figure 8.6 depicts a light ray as it passes from air into a container of water. Different media have different speeds of propagation, so light travels at different speeds through different media. Which way light will refract relative to normal depends on whether the wave is transitioning to a faster or slower medium. As a wave moves from one medium into an optically denser medium (from a faster medium to a slower medium), the wave

bends toward the normal. As a wave moves from a medium into an optically less dense medium (from a slower medium to a faster medium), the wave bends away from the normal.

The mathematic relationship for this behavior is called *Snell's law,* which is expressed mathematically as follows, where n = the index of refraction and θ = the angle of refraction.

$$n_1 \sin\theta_1 = n_2 \sin\theta_2$$

The index of refraction is a ratio of the speed of light in a vacuum to the speed of light in a given material. This mathematic relationship is expressed as follows, where c = the speed of light in a vacuum (3×10^8 m/s) and v_s = the speed of light in a given substance.

$$n = \frac{c}{v_s}$$

SAMPLE PROBLEM

13. If the index of refraction for acrylic is 1.490, what is the speed of light in acrylic?
    A. 2.01×10^8 m/s
    B. 4.38×10^8 m/s
    C. 1.25×10^8 m/s
    D. 0.489×10^8 m/s

Answer

A—To determine the speed of light in acrylic, divide the speed of light by index of refraction for acrylic. Using the following equation, the speed of light in acrylic is determined to be 2.01×10^8 m/s.

$$n = \frac{c}{v_s}$$

Convert the equation to solve for speed of light in a substance (v_s).

$$v_s = \frac{3 \times 10^8}{1.490}$$

$$v_s = 2.01 \times 10^8 \text{ m/s}$$

Optics

The previous discussion of reflection assumed a plane mirror. However, the shape of the mirror, specifically with spherical mirrors (i.e., convex or concave), changes the direction of reflection. Concave mirrors have positive focal lengths, whereas convex mirrors have negative focal lengths. Concave mirrors form a variety of image shapes, sizes, and orientations, depending on the focal length of the mirror and where the object is placed. Figure 8.7 depicts a concave mirror with the focal point (f) and curvature (C). With the object beyond the center of curvature (C), we have an image that is smaller than the object and inverted in orientation. If we place the object at C, the resulting image is the same size as the object and inverted in orientation. If the object is between C and the focal point (f), the image is larger than the object and inverted in orientation. If the object is at f, there is no image formed. If the object is between f and the mirror, the image is upright and larger in size and virtual. Convex mirrors can form only images that are smaller and upright. Real images are always inverted, and virtual images are always upright.

Lenses form images by refraction. There are two basic types of lenses: convex (converging) and concave (diverging). Convex lenses always have positive focal lengths, and concave lenses always have negative focal lengths. Convex lenses can form a variety of image shapes, sizes, and orientations, depending on the focal length of the lens and the object's position. When an object is placed at a position greater than $2f$, the image is reduced, inverted, and on the opposite side of the lens. The placement of an object at $2f$ results in an image that is the same size as the object, inverted, and on the opposite side of the lens. The placement of an object between $2f$ and f results in an image that is larger than the object, inverted, and on the opposite side of the lens. When the object is placed at f, no image is formed. If the object is between f and the lens, the image is upright, larger, and on the same side of the lens. A concave lens can form only an image that is upright and smaller than the object.

Atomic Structure

Many discussions of physical principles are aided by an understanding of basic atomic structure. The atom is composed of three fundamental particles: protons, neutrons, and electrons (Fig. 8.8). Protons are one part of the nucleus of the atom and carry one unit of positive electric charge. Neutrons are the other principal part of the nucleus and are electrically neutral. Electrons orbit the nucleus in specific energy levels and carry one unit of negative electric charge. The energy levels or shells in which the electrons orbit are lettered beginning with "k" (i.e., k, l, m, n, o, etc.). The closer the electron shell, the stronger the **binding energy** (how tightly the electron is bound to the nucleus). Each shell holds a specific number of electrons. This number may be found using the following formula, where n is the shell number (k = 1, l = 2, m = 3, and so on):

$$2n^2$$

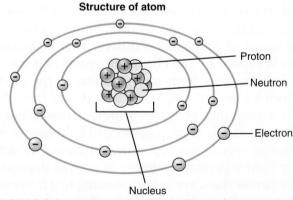

Structure of atom

FIGURE 8.8   Basic atomic structure. (From Johnston JN, Fauber TL: *Essentials of radiographic physics and imaging*, ed 2, St Louis, 2016, Elsevier Mosby.)

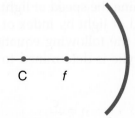

C   f

FIGURE 8.7   Concave mirror.

When the number of positive charges (protons in the nucleus) equals the number of negative charges (electrons in orbit), the atom is said to be stable.

The Nature of Electricity

The electric property of a given material depends on the nature of its atoms. Materials whose atoms have loosely bound **valence electrons** (electrons in the outermost shell) are good conductors of electricity. Conversely, materials whose valence electrons are tightly bound are good electric insulators. Because the protons (positive charges) of an atom are tightly bound in the nucleus of the atom and not free to move about, most discussions of the flow of electricity involve negative charges (electrons).

Coulomb's Law

There are two types of basic electric charge, positive and negative. The smallest unit of positive charge rests with the proton and the smallest unit of negative charge rests with the electron. Like charges will repel each other, whereas opposite charges will attract. This force of attraction or repulsion is expressed by Coulomb's law, which states that the force of attraction or repulsion between two charged objects is directly proportional to the product of their quantities and inversely proportional to the square of the distance between them. The unit of measure for electric charge is the coulomb. The force of attraction or repulsion is determined by the mathematic relationship expressed by Coulomb's law, where k = a constant (9×10^9 N-m^2/C^2), q_1 and q_2 = the charges on objects 1 and 2 expressed in coulombs, and r = the distance between the two charged objects in meters.

$$F = \frac{kq_1q_2}{r^2}$$

SAMPLE PROBLEM

14. An object of charge 25 μC is placed 67 cm from an object of charge 50 μC. What is the magnitude of the resulting force bewteen the two objects?
    A. 17.28 N
    B. 28.53 N
    C. 1.73×10^{13} N
    D. 8.64×10^{12} N

Answer

B—To solve this problem use Coulomb's law. First, convert μC to C, remembering that 1 μC is 1×10^{-6} C, and convert the distance from centimeters to meters. After insertion of the correct values into the equation, remembering to square the distance (r^2), the force between the two objects is determined to be 28.53 N.

$$F = \frac{kq_1q_2}{r^2}$$

$$F = \frac{\left(9 \times 10^9 \ N - m^2/C^2\right)\left(50 \times 10^{-6} \ C\right)\left(25 \times 10^{-6} \ C\right)}{\left(0.67 \ m\right)^2}$$

$$F = 28.53 \ N$$

Electric Fields

An electric field exists around charged objects. This field force created by the charged object is basically a change in the space that surrounds the charged object. One way to test the nature of this electric field is to use a positive test charge. If the electric field is generated by a negative charge, the test charge will experience an attractive force. If the electric field is generated by a positive charge, the test charge will experience a repulsive force. Owing to these interactions, scientists have defined the direction of an electric field to be away from a positive charge and toward a negative charge. The magnitude of an electric field is stated mathematically as follows, where E = the magnitude of the electric field, F = the force a test charge would experience, and q_o = the magnitude of the test charge.

$$E = \frac{F}{q_o}$$

Because electric fields are vector quantities, they should be treated as such. The direction of an electric field is defined as the direction a positive test charge would be moved when placed in the electric field.

15. An electric field of magnitude 280,000 N/C points due east at a certain spot. What are the magnitude and direction of the force that acts on a charge of –10 μC?
    A. 2.8 N to the west
    B. 2.8 N to the east
    C. 28 N to the west
    D. 28 N to the east

Answer

A—To determine the magnitude of the force *(F)* acting on the charge, multiply the magnitude of the electric field *(E)* by the magnitude of the test charge *(q₀)*. Because the charge is negative, it acts opposite to the direction of the electric field. After insertion of the appropriate values in the electric field equation, the magnitude of the charge is determined to be 2.8 N to the west.

$$E = \frac{F}{q_o}$$

Convert the equation to solve for the force *(F)* the test charge will experience:

$$F = Eq_o$$

$$F = (280,000 \text{ N/C})(-10 \text{ μC})$$

Remember that 1 μC is 1×10^{-6} C.

$$F = (280,000 \text{ N/C})(-10 \text{ μC})$$

$$F = (280,000 \text{ N/C})(-0.00001 \text{ C})$$

$$F = -2.8 \text{ N}$$

The negative sign in the answer indicates the direction of the force relative to the electric field.

$$F = 2.8 \text{ N to the west}$$

Nature and Properties of Circuits

An electric circuit is basically a series of electronic devices or circuit elements connected by a conductive wire that allows electric charges to continuously flow. For continuous flow to exist, there must be a conductive pathway from the positive terminal to the negative terminal and there must be a potential difference between the terminals.

The flow of current is determined by the voltage available and the resistance of the circuit. The mathematic relationship between voltage, current, and resistance is known as *Ohm's law*, which states that the potential difference (voltage) in a circuit or any part of that circuit is equal to the current (amperes) multiplied by the resistance (ohms). Ohm's law is expressed as follows, where *V* = potential difference in voltage expressed in volts, *I* = current expressed in amperes, and *R* = resistance expressed in ohms.

$$V = IR$$

Voltage is an expression of the potential difference between two points and is measured in volts. A volt is the work (in joules) that may be done per unit of charge. Current is measured in amperes, which is defined as one coulomb of electricity flowing by a given point in one second. Resistance is measured in ohms and is that property of a circuit element that impedes the flow of electricity. One ohm is equal to the resistance between two points necessary to allow a current of one ampere when one volt is applied.

There are two types of basic circuits: series circuits and parallel circuits. A series circuit has only one pathway through which current can flow, so current is the same through all resistors. A parallel circuit has several pathways through which current can flow, but all resistors are connected directly to the same battery, so the voltage supplied for each resistor is the same. To determine the total resistance of a series circuit, you would add the individual resistors. To determine the total resistance of a parallel circuit, you would add the reciprocal of the individual resistors and then take the reciprocal of that value. Once the total resistance is determined and the type of circuit used is known, the current flowing through each resistor can be determined.

16. A circuit consists of a 5-ohm resistor, a 10-ohm resistor, and a 15-ohm resistor. The resistors are placed in series and then wired to a 75-V power supply. Determine the current flowing in the circuit.
    A. 0.5 amp
    B. 2.5 amp

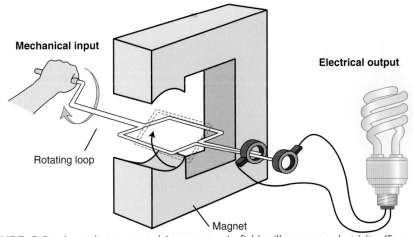

FIGURE 8.9 A conductor rotated in a magnetic field will generate electricity. (From Johnston JN, Fauber TL: *Essentials of radiographic physics and imaging,* ed 2, St Louis, 2016, Elsevier Mosby.)

C. 10.0 amp

D. 4.0 amp

Answer

B—Before the current flowing through the circuit can be determined, the total resistance must be calculated. Because the resistors are placed in a series, the total resistance is determined by adding the values of the individual resistors.

$$\text{Total Resistance}_{(\text{in a series})} = R1 + R2 + R3$$

$$\text{Total Resistance}_{(\text{in a series})} = 5\ \text{ohm} +$$
$$10\ \text{ohm} + 15\ \text{ohm}$$

$$\text{Total Resistance}_{(\text{in a series})} = 30\ \text{ohm}$$

To determine the current in the circuit, use the Ohm's law equation. After insertion of the appropriate values into the equation, the current flowing in the circuit is determined to be 2.5 amp.

$$V = IR$$

Convert the equation to solve for current *(I)*.

$$I = \frac{75\ \text{volts}}{30\ \text{ohms}}$$

$$I = 2.5\ \text{amps}$$

Magnetism and Electricity

Magnetism is that property of a material that will attract iron, cobalt, or nickel. Magnetic fields exist as lines of force in space known as *flux.* These flux lines create elliptical loops in space that extend from the north pole externally to the south pole of the magnet. As with electric charges, like magnetic poles repel each other and opposite magnetic poles attract. Additionally, the force of attraction or repulsion between two magnetic fields varies directly as the strength of the magnetic poles and inversely as the square of the distance between them. The strength of a magnetic field is measured in Teslas.

Electricity and magnetism are two parts of the same basic force known as electromagnetism. That is, any flow of electricity, whether in space or in a conductor, will create an associated magnetic field around it. Likewise, any moving magnetic field will create an electric current. This induction of an electric current is known as *electromagnetic induction.* When a conductor is passed back and forth in a magnetic field or the flux from a moving magnetic field passes through a conductor, an electric current will be induced to flow in that conductor. Figure 8.9 demonstrates a conductor being rotated in a magnetic field that induces current in the loop to power the light bulb.

HESI Hint

Magnetism and electricity are fundamental to x-ray production. There is no magical process involved in the production of x-rays by medical imaging equipment. It is simply the manipulation of electricity.

POSTTEST

1. Select the word that means the same as the underlined word in the sentence. The doctor gave a <u>concise</u> explanation of the treatment plan.
   A. Slow but informative
   B. Hasty and incomplete
   C. Long and detailed
   D. Brief but clear

2. Select the words for the blanks that make this sentence grammatically correct. Sam cooked dinner for _____ and _____.
   A. him, me
   B. him, I
   C. he, I
   D. he, me

3. How does a catalyst increase the rate of a chemical reaction?
   A. Increases the temperature
   B. Increases the concentration
   C. Reduces the activation energy
   D. Reduces the surface area

Change fraction to decimal:
4. $\frac{5}{16} =$ _____
   A. 0.50
   B. 0.60
   C. 0.3125
   D. 0.4165

Change fraction to decimal:
5. $\frac{5}{8} =$ _____
   A. 1.11
   B. 0.625
   C. 0.375
   D. 1.60

6. Which word in the sentence is an adverb? She suddenly felt as if someone was watching her.
   A. suddenly
   B. felt
   C. was
   D. watching

7. A classroom consists of three girls and six boys. One student will be randomly selected to pass out the assignments. What is the probability that a girl will be selected?
   A. 33%
   B. 40%
   C. 50%
   D. 66%

8. Select the best definition of the word *exacerbate*.
   A. To expel urine
   B. To expel feces
   C. To increase in size
   D. To make worse

9. Which is a characteristic of a high-energy wave?
   A. Low amplitude
   B. Low frequency
   C. Short wavelength
   D. Slow speed

10. Which sentence contains a proper noun?
    A. We went to the zoo to see the animals.
    B. I've never been to London before.
    C. The mayor arrived in time for the parade.
    D. The general's army traveled south.

11. One length of rope is 3.5 feet long and another is 4.2 feet long. How many feet longer is the second length of rope than the first?
    A. 0.7
    B. 0.8
    C. 1.2
    D. 1.7

12. Which is an imperative sentence?
    A. Oh, I can't believe you did that.
    B. How dare you!
    C. Who do you think you are?
    D. Please go away.

13. Which occurs during cytokinesis?
    A. Two daughter cells are formed.
    B. The nuclear envelope breaks down.
    C. Chromosomes align across the middle of the cell.
    D. Chromatids separate and migrate to opposite poles.

14. Select the meaning of the underlined word in the sentence.
    The patient's abnormal posture is due to a congenital condition.
    A. Related to an unknown cause
    B. Present from birth
    C. Lasting a long time
    D. Of sudden onset

15. Sixteen high school students completed a math exam, but only 12 students received a passing grade. Which expression represents the ratio of passing grades to failing grades?
    A. 5:4
    B. 4:1
    C. 3:4
    D. 3:1

16. Select the best word for the blank in the following sentence. The prize money was divided _____ the winning team.
    A. between
    B. among
    C. throughout
    D. over

17. The initial speed of a go-kart is 12 miles/second (m/s). After 8 seconds, the go-kart achieves a speed of 24 m/s. What is the magnitude of acceleration?
    A. $1.5 \, \text{m/s}^2$
    B. $4.5 \, \text{m/s}^2$
    C. $12 \, \text{m/s}^2$
    D. $24 \, \text{m/s}^2$

18. Chromosomes align across the center of the cell during which phase of mitosis?
    A. Anaphase
    B. Telophase
    C. Metaphase
    D. Prophase

19. A patient has a history of back pain that has been recurring for several years. Which term best describes this pain?
    A. Paroxysmal
    B. Residual
    C. Chronic
    D. Labile

20. Which reproductive process begins with two haploid cells and ends with four haploid cells?
    A. Meiosis I
    B. Meiosis II
    C. Mitosis
    D. Binary fission

21. Which term describes the process in which a DNA template is used to create a complementary RNA molecule?
    A. Translation
    B. Replication
    C. Duplication
    D. Transcription

22. Which word in this sentence is an indirect object? The professor gave Tim the book to read at home.
    A. professor
    B. Tim
    C. book
    D. home

23. Which statement uses a euphemism?
    A. Bill had to be let go because he was always late for work.
    B. Dave looked pale as a ghost when he heard the news.
    C. The coach's bark was worse than his bite.
    D. We are all grateful for the brave firemen that serve our city.

24. Which is the end result of DNA translation?
    A. Synthesis of proteins
    B. Formation of a DNA template
    C. Synthesis of mRNA
    D. Formation of identical DNA molecules

25. Which determines the mass number of an element?
    A. Mass of protons and electrons
    B. Mass of neutrons and electrons
    C. Average mass of that element's isotopes
    D. Number of protons and neutrons

26. Which area of the heart's electrical conduction system triggers the sequence that results in a normal cardiac rhythm?
    A. Bundle of His
    B. Atrioventricular node
    C. Sinoatrial node
    D. Purkinje fibers

27. If a DNA strand has a base sequence GTACGT, what is the sequence of the complementary segment of DNA?
    A. GTACGT
    B. CATGCA
    C. TGCATG
    D. ACGTAC

28. Thirty-six (36) grams of carbon-12 is equal to how many moles?
    A. 1
    B. 2
    C. 3
    D. 4

29. Which bones are part of the axial skeleton?
    A. Femurs
    B. Clavicles
    C. Vertebrae
    D. Scapulae

30. Which type of radiation is classified as electromagnetic?
    A. Positron
    B. Alpha
    C. Beta
    D. Gamma

31. Only half of the boys at summer camp went on the canoe trip. Eight girls also went on the canoe trip. The total number of campers who went on the canoe trip was 14. What is the total number of boys who attended summer camp?
    A. 8
    B. 10
    C. 12
    D. 14

32. What gland produces hormones responsible for regulating the amount of glucose in the blood?
    A. Adrenal
    B. Thyroid
    C. Pituitary
    D. Pancreas

33. A patient's ankle is red, swollen, and feels warm to touch. Which term best describes the patient's ankle?
    A. Inflamed
    B. Distended
    C. Obtunded
    D. Flushed

34. What is the main function of Schwann cells in the peripheral nervous system?
    A. Amplify the nerve signal along the axon
    B. Increase the speed of nerve conduction
    C. Regulate all nerve cell functions
    D. Receive stimuli from other nerve cells

35. It takes a car 2 minutes to travel 1,200 meters. What is the average speed of the car in meters per second (m/sec)?
    A. 10 m/sec
    B. 60 m/sec
    C. 100 m/sec
    D. 600 m/sec

36. What happens during an oxidation reaction?
   A. Gain of hydrogen
   B. Gain of electrons
   C. Loss of oxygen
   D. Loss of electrons

37. A rock is kicked from the top of a building that is 44.1 m tall. If the rock travels at a speed of 8.6 m/sec, how far from the building will the rock land?
   A. 8.6 m
   B. 17.2 m
   C. 25.8 m
   D. 73.96 m

38. Urine passes outside of the body through which structure?
   A. Ureter
   B. Urethra
   C. Bladder
   D. Renal tubule

39. What is 6:30 PM in military time?
   A. 2030
   B. 0630
   C. 1430
   D. 1830

40. A commercial airplane has a mass of 80,000 kilograms and travels at a maximum speed of 900 kilometers/hour. What is the kinetic energy of the airplane at maximum speed?
   A. 3024×10^{10} J
   B. 10.71 J
   C. 29.8 J
   D. 2.5×10^6 J

41. Which type of neurons detect changes in blood pressure?
   A. Nociceptors
   B. Baroreceptors
   C. Proprioceptors
   D. Chemoreceptors

42. Which is the strongest type of chemical bond?
   A. Ionic
   B. Dipole-dipole
   C. Hydrogen
   D. Covalent

43. A patient is diagnosed with a subcutaneous tumor. Where is the tumor located?
   A. Around the spinal cord
   B. Under the tongue
   C. Beneath the skin
   D. Inside the abdomen

44. A circuit consisting of two 10-ohm resistors and a 25-ohm resistor is placed in a series. How much voltage is needed to provide 4 amps of current?
   A. 2.2 V
   B. 11.25 V
   C. 140 V
   D. 180 V

Use the Passage below to Answer Questions 45-50.

Jonas Salk

Jonas Salk was an American physician and one of the leading medical researchers of the twentieth century. He is famous for creating the first safe and effective vaccine for polio, a highly infectious incurable disease that was responsible for thousands of cases of paralysis each year in the United States.

Salk received degrees in science and medicine before taking a position as the director of the Virus Research Laboratory at the University of Pittsburgh in 1947. By this time, polio was one of the most feared diseases of the twentieth century. Polio, a highly infectious disease caused by the poliovirus, can cause paralysis of muscles in the limbs, throat, and chest. Polio can lead to death when the muscles responsible for breathing become paralyzed.

By 1951, Salk developed a vaccine made of a "killed" polio virus. The vaccine was produced from polio viruses that had been grown in a laboratory and then destroyed. When the "killed virus" was injected into the bloodstream, Salk reasoned that the vaccine would trick the immune system into producing anti-polio antibodies. Salk also believed that his vaccine could immunize patients without risk of infection.

Early testing of Salk's polio vaccine began in 1952, when children at two institutions were injected with the vaccine. (Salk also tested the vaccine on himself, his wife, and his three sons.) All of the test subjects developed anti-polio antibodies and did not experience any negative reactions to the vaccine. About 1.8 million children would eventually receive the vaccine during the test phase. At the height of the polio epidemic in 1952, there were more than 57,000 cases reported in the United States. A decade later, that number fell to less than one thousand.

By the time the vaccine was approved for use, Jonas Salk was a medical celebrity and a national hero. In 1955, Salk received a special citation from President Dwight D. Eisenhower at a ceremony held in the Rose Garden at the White House. Having developed the vaccine that would lead to the eradication of polio in the United States, Salk will always be remembered as one of the greatest medical pioneers of the twentieth century.

45. Which is the best summary of the passage?
    A. Jonas Salk created the first successful polio vaccine. He developed a vaccine made of a "killed" polio virus. After the vaccine was approved for public use, the number of new cases of polio began to decline rapidly. Salk would be considered a national hero for stopping polio.
    B. Jonas Salk created the first safe and effective polio vaccine. He tested the vaccine by injecting live poliovirus into his test subjects. Within a decade of initial testing, the number of polio cases had decreased dramatically. Today he is known as the man who cured polio.
    C. Jonas Salk was a famous medical researcher. He discovered the poliovirus in 1947 and began working on a cure. By 1951, he developed a vaccine that was able to trick the body into developing antibodies to kill the virus. When the vaccine proved to be effective, he became a celebrity.
    D. Jonas Salk was a famous American physician who created a vaccine for the poliovirus. In 1952, the vaccine was tested on children with polio. All the children developed antibodies and there were no negative reactions to the vaccine. He became a hero for ending polio in the United States.

46. Which is **not** a detail from the passage?
    A. Salk was the director of a virus research laboratory in Pittsburgh.
    B. Salk received a citation from the President of the United States.
    C. Salk gave the vaccine to himself before it was tested on children.
    D. Salk earned degrees in science and medicine before 1947.

47. Which describes the purpose of the polio vaccine?
    A. It helps reduce the symptoms of polio.
    B. It makes the body immune to the poliovirus.
    C. It destroys the poliovirus within the body.
    D. It cures people who have polio.

48. According to the passage, why was Jonas Salk considered a national hero?
    A. He discovered the poliovirus.
    B. He created a vaccine for polio.
    C. He developed a cure for polio.
    D. He founded a polio research laboratory.

49. What is the main purpose of the passage?
    A. To explain why Jonas Salk is an important figure
    B. To trace the stages of development of the polio vaccine
    C. To describe how polio affected the United States population
    D. To describe how Jonas Salk invented a cure for polio

50. What does the word "negative" mean as it is used in the fourth paragraph?
    A. Normal
    B. Absent
    C. Harmful
    D. Less than zero

ANSWERS TO POSTTEST

1. D
2. A—Objective case pronouns are required to complete this sentence. The pronouns "him" and "me" are objects of the preposition "for."
3. C
4. C
5. B
6. A
7. A
8. D
9. C
10. B—A proper noun is the official name of a person, place, or thing. London is a proper noun.
11. A
12. D—An imperative sentence makes a command or request. Option D is an imperative sentence.
13. A
14. B
15. D
16. B
17. A
18. C
19. C
20. B
21. D
22. B

23. A
24. A
25. D
26. C
27. B
28. C
29. C
30. D
31. C
32. D
33. A
34. B
35. A
36. D
37. C
38. B
39. D
40. A
41. B
42. D
43. C
44. D
45. A
46. C
47. B
48. B
49. A
50. C

GLOSSARY

A

Abstract noun: The name of a quality or a general idea (e.g., persistence, democracy).

Acceleration: The rate of change in velocity over a period of time.

Acid: A compound that is a hydrogen or proton donor. It is corrosive to metals, changes blue litmus paper red, and becomes less acidic when mixed with bases.

Adjective: A word, phrase, or clause that modifies a noun (the *biology* book) or pronoun (He is *nice*.).

Adverb: A word, phrase, or clause that modifies a verb, an adjective, or another adverb.

Alleles: Alternate versions of a gene.

Amino acids: Organic compounds that contain at least one amino group and a carboxyl group; building blocks of proteins.

Amylase: Enzyme that begins digestion of complex carbohydrates; secreted by the salivary glands and the pancreas.

Anatomic position: Provides a baseline reference point for areas of the body. In this position, the body is erect, the feet are slightly apart, the head is held high, the arms are at the sides, and the palms of the hands are facing forward.

Anterior: Directional term meaning toward the front.

Antonym: A word that means the opposite of another word.

Appendicular skeleton: The part of the skeleton that includes the shoulder and hip girdles, and the extremities.

Atom: The basic building block of a molecule, which contains a nucleus and orbits.

Atomic mass: The mass of a single element; approximately equal to mass number.

Atomic number: The number of protons in the nucleus, and it defines an atom of a particular element.

Atomic weight: The *average* mass of each of an element's isotopes.

Autonomic nervous system: Division of the peripheral nervous system which controls functions such as digestion, force and rate of heart contraction, blood pressure, and diameter. The two divisions of the autonomic nervous system are the *parasympathetic division* ("rest and digest") and the *sympathetic division* ("fight or flight").

Average speed: The distance an object travels divided by the time the object travels without regard to direction of travel.

Axial skeleton: Consists of the skull, vertebral column, twelve pairs of ribs, and sternum.

B

Base: A hydrogen or proton acceptor and generally has a hydroxide (OH) group in the makeup of the molecule. Bases are also called *alkaline compounds* and are substances that denature proteins, making them feel very slick; they change red litmus paper blue and become less basic when mixed with acids.

Basic unit of measure: Standard unit of a system by which a quantity is accounted for and expressed (grams, liters, or meters).

Binary fission: Type of asexual reproduction; parent cell splits into two identical daughter cells.

Binding energy: How tightly the electron is bound to the nucleus.

Biochemistry: The study of chemical processes in living organisms.

Brainstem: Part of the brain that is continuous with the spinal cord; controls many vital functions such as respiration and heart rate.

C

Catalysts: Substances that accelerate a reaction by reducing the activation energy or the amount of energy necessary for a reaction to occur.

Cell: The basic unit of life and the building block of tissues and organs.

Celsius: A temperature system used in most of the world and by the scientific community; abbreviated C. It has these characteristics: zero degrees (0° C) is the freezing point of pure water at sea level, and 100° C is the boiling point of pure water at sea level. Most people have a body temperature of 37° C.

Centripetal acceleration: Rotational motion equivalent of acceleration.

Cerebellum: The part of the brain responsible for muscular coordination.

Cerebrum: The part of the brain associated with sensory interpretation, movement, thinking, and personality.

Chemical equations: Combination of elements or compounds called reactants responding to create a product or end result. Equations are expressed in the following ways: Reactants → Products; Reactants ← Products; Reactants ↔ Products.

Chromosomes: Compact, rod-shaped bodies located within the nucleus of a cell; contain DNA.

Clause: A group of words that has a subject and a predicate.

Cliché: An expression or idea that has lost its originality or impact over time because of excessive use.

Codon: Three-base sequence of messenger RNA.

Collective noun: A collective noun is a noun that represents a group of persons, animals, or things (e.g., family, flock, furniture).

Combustion: A self-sustaining exothermic chemical reaction usually initiated by heat acting on oxygen and a fuel compound such as hydrocarbons.

Common denominator: Two or more fractions having the same denominator.

Common noun: A common noun is the general, not the particular, name of a person, place, or thing (e.g., nurse, hospital, syringe).

Compound: The combination of two or more elements or atoms.

Compound sentence: A sentence that has two or more independent clauses. Each independent clause has a subject and a predicate and can stand alone as a sentence.

Conjunction: A word that joins words, phrases, or clauses.

Connotation: The emotions or feelings that the reader attaches to words.

Constant: A number that cannot change.

Context clue: The information provided in the words or sentences surrounding an unknown word or words.

Covalent bond: Two atoms share electrons, generally in pairs, one from each atom.

Cytology: The study of cells.

D

Declarative: A declarative sentence makes a statement.

Decomposition: A chemical reaction often described as the opposite of synthesis because it is the breaking of a compound into its component parts.

Deep: Further into the body.

Denominator: The bottom number in a fraction.

Deoxyribonucleic acid (DNA): A unique molecule specific to a particular organism; it contains the genetic code that is necessary for replication.

Deoxyribose: A sugar used in the formation of DNA.

Dependent clause: A dependent clause begins with a subordinating conjunction and does not express a complete thought and therefore cannot stand alone as a sentence.

Dermis: Deep layer of skin that is connective tissue with blood vessels, nerve endings, and the associated skin structures.

Diencephalon: The part of the brain that contains the thalamus which routes incoming sensory information to the appropriate part of the cerebrum, and the hypothalamus which monitors many of the conditions of the body, controls the autonomic nervous system, and interacts with the endocrine system.

Digit: Any number from 0 through 9 (e.g., the number 7 is a digit).

Direct object: The person or thing that is directly affected by the action of the verb.

Distal: Directional term that refers to farther away from the point of attachment of an extremity to the trunk.

Dividend: The number being divided.

Divisor: The number by which the dividend is divided.

Double replacement: A reaction that involves two ionic compounds. The positive ion from one compound combines with the negative ion of the other compound. The result is two new ionic compounds that have "switched partners."

E

Electron: A structure in an atom that is at the outermost part of the atom and has a negative charge. Electrons orbit the nucleus at fantastic speeds, forming electron clouds.

Electron clouds: The group of electrons revolving around the nucleus of an atom; a cloudlike group of electrons.

Electron transport chain: Series of steps in cellular respiration that produces water and ATP.

Epidermis: Superficial layer of skin that made of dead, keratinized epithelial cells.

Equilibrium: A state in which reactants are forming products at the same rate that products are forming reactants.

Erythrocytes: Red blood cells.

Euphemism: A mild, indirect, or vague term that has been substituted for one that is considered harsh, blunt, or offensive.

Exclamatory: A sentence expressing strong feelings or making an exclamation.

Exponent: A number or symbol placed above and after another number or symbol (a superscript or subscript), indicating the number of times to multiply.

Expression: A mathematic sentence containing constants and variables (e.g., $3x - 2$).

External respiration: The exchange of gases between the atmosphere and the blood through the alveoli.

F

Factor: A number that divides evenly into another number.

Fahrenheit: A temperature-measuring system used only in the United States, its territories, Belize, and Jamaica; abbreviated F. It is rarely used for any scientific measurements except for body temperature. It has these characteristics: zero degrees ($0°$) is the freezing point of sea water or heavy brine at sea level; $32°$ F is the freezing point of pure water at sea level; $212°$ F is the boiling point of pure water at sea level; most people have a body temperature of $98.6°$ F.

Force: A push or pull on an object.

Fraction bar: The line between the numerator and denominator. The bar is another symbol for division.

Friction: A force that opposes motion and is expressed in newtons.

G

Glycolysis: Anaerobic breakdown of glucose; first stage in cell respiration.

Golgi apparatus: Cell organelle that packages, processes, and distributes molecules about or from the cell.

Groups: Elements that are placed together in columns in the periodic table.

H

Hemopoiesis: Blood cell formation.

Heterozygous: Trait in an organism that contains different alleles.

Histology: The study of tissues.

Homozygous: Trait in an organism that contains identical alleles.

I

Imperative: An imperative sentence makes a command or request.

Impulse equation: When both sides of Newton's second law of motion are multiplied by Δt (change in time), a new relationship between force and time is established ($F\Delta t = m\Delta v$) because a force applied over a period of time is an impulse.

Independent clause: An independent clause expresses a complete thought and can stand alone as a sentence.

Indirect object: The person or thing that is indirectly affected by the action of the verb.

Inference: An educated guess or conclusion drawn by the reader based on the available facts and information.

Inferior: Directional term meaning below.

Interjection: A word or phrase that expresses emotion or exclamation.

Internal respiration: The exchange of gases between the blood and the body cells.

Interphase: Stage of the cell cycle during which growth and DNA synthesis occur.

Interrogative: An interrogative sentence asks a question.

Ionic bond: An electrostatic attraction between two oppositely charged ions or a cation and an anion. This type of bond is generally formed between a metal (cation) and a nonmetal (anion).

Isotope: Different kinds of the same atom that vary in weight; for a given element, the number of protons remains the same, while the number of neutrons varies to make the different isotopes.

J

Joule: A newton-meter or a kilogram-meter squared per second squared (kg-m^2/s^2).

K

Kelvin: A unit of measure for temperature that is used only in the scientific community. Kelvin (K) has these characteristics: zero degrees Kelvin (0K) is $-273°$ C and is thought to be the lowest temperature achievable or absolute zero (0); the freezing point of water is 273K; the boiling point of water is 373K; most people have a body temperature of 310K.

Kinetic energy: The energy resulting from the motion of the object that is represented by the following equation, where KE = kinetic energy, m = mass of the object, and v = velocity.

Krebs cycle: Series of reactions that occur in the mitochondrion during cellular respiration.

L

Lateral: Directional term meaning away from the midline.

Law of universal gravitation: Every object in the universe attracts every other object in the universe.

Least common denominator: The smallest multiple that two numbers share.

Leukocytes: White blood cells.

M

Mass number: The combined number of protons and neutrons in an element.

Mathematic sign: A symbol used in mathematics. A mathematic sign makes up one of the three parts of scientific notation and designates whether the number is positive or negative (+ or −).

Medial: Directional term meaning toward the midline.

Meiosis: The special cell division that takes place in the gonads (ovaries and testes) as part of sexual reproduction. In the process, the chromosome number is reduced from 46 to 23, so when the egg and the sperm unite in fertilization, the zygote will have the correct number of chromosomes.

Messenger RNA (mRNA): Type of RNA formed from a template of DNA; carries coded information to form proteins.

Metabolic pathway: Series of linked chemical reactions.

Metaphase plate: Disk formed during metaphase in which the chromosomes align on equatorial plane of the cell.

Misplaced modifiers: Words or groups of words that are not located properly in relation to the words they modify.

Mitosis: The process in which the DNA is duplicated and distributed evenly to two identical daughter cells. Phases include prophase, prometaphase, metaphase, anaphase, and telophase.

Mole: A way to express concentrations of atoms. It is 6.02×10^{23} of particles.

Momentum: The amount of motion displayed by an object and is represented by the mathematic equation p = mΔv, where p = the momentum in kilogram-meters per second, m = the mass in kilograms, and Δv = the change in velocity of the object.

N

Nephrons: The functional units of the kidneys that filter wastes out of the blood.

Neuroglia: Connective tissue cells that support neurons.

Neutron: Part of the nucleus of an atom that has no charge.

Newton: Unit of force.

Noun: A word or group of words that names a person, place, thing, or idea.

Nucleus: The positively charged mass within an atom, composed of neutrons and protons, and possessing most of the mass but occupying only a small fraction of the volume of the atom.

Numerator: The top number in a fraction.

O

Orbit: The outermost part of the atom that consists of electrons that spin around the nucleus at fantastic speeds forming electron clouds.

Organelles: Any of many cell "organs" or organized components.

Osteoblasts: Cells that form bone tissue.

Osteoclasts: Cells that break down bone tissue.

P

Parallel circuit: A circuit with several pathways through which current can flow, but all resistors are connected directly to the same battery, so the voltage supplied for each resistor is the same.

Participial phrase: A phrase that is formed by a participle, its object, and the object's modifiers; the participial phrase functions as an adjective.

Participle: A type of verb form that functions as an adjective.

Percent: Per hundred (part per hundred).

Periodic table: A table that organizes the elements based on their structure and thus helps predict the properties of each of the elements. It is made up of a series of rows called *periods* and columns called *groups*.

Periods: A series of rows within the periodic table that classify the elements.

Personal pronoun: A personal pronoun refers to a specific person, place, thing, or idea by indicating the person speaking (first person), the person or people spoken to (second person), or any other person, place, thing, or idea being talked about (third person).

pH: The concentrations of acids. The pH scale commonly in use ranges from 0 to 14 and is a measure of the acidity or alkalinity of a solution.

Phagocytosis: Process in which cells engulf food particles through the cell membrane.

Phospholipids: Phosphate-containing fat molecules; form the bilayer of a cell membrane.

Photosynthesis: Chemical process that converts light energy to synthesize carbohydrates.

Phrase: A group of two or more words that acts as a single part of speech in a sentence.

Place value: The value of the position of a digit in a number (e.g., in the number 659, the number 5 is in the "tens" position).

Planes: Imaginary flat plates along which cuts, either real or virtual, can be made. Types of planes include sagittal, midsagittal, frontal (coronal), and transverse (horizontal).

Possessive pronoun: A form of personal pronoun that shows possession or ownership.

Posterior: Directional term meaning toward the back.

Potential energy: The energy the object has because of its position and is expressed by the equation PE = mgh, where PE = potential energy, m = mass of the object, g = acceleration caused by gravity, and h = the height at which the object is located above the ground.

Predicate: The part of the sentence that tells what the subject does or what is done to the subject.

Predicate adjective: An adjective that follows a linking verb and helps to explain the subject.

Predicate nominative: A noun or pronoun that follows a linking verb and helps to explain or rename the subject.

Prefix: Each metric measurement is composed of a metric prefix and a basic unit of measure (e.g., "kilogram," where "kilo" is the prefix and "gram" is the basic unit of measure). The prefixes are the same and have the same meaning or value, regardless of which basic unit of measurement (grams, liters, or meters) is used. Prefixes are the quantifiers of the measurement units. All of the prefixes are based on multiples of ten. Any one of the prefixes can be combined with one of the basic units of measurement.

Preposition: A word that shows the relationship of a noun or pronoun to some other word in the sentence.

Product: The answer to a multiplication problem.

Products: Substances or compounds created from a chemical reaction.

Projectile: An object that displays two types of motion simultaneously.

Pronoun: A word that takes the place of a noun, another pronoun, or a group of words acting as a noun.

Proper noun: A proper noun is the official name of a person, place, or thing (e.g., Fred, Paris, Washington University). Proper nouns are capitalized.

Proportion: Two ratios that have equal values.

Proton: Part of the nucleus of an atom that has a positive electric charge.

Proximal: Directional term meaning closer to the point of attachment of the extremity to the trunk.

Punnett square: Grid used to predict genotype and phenotype of the offspring of sexual reproduction.

Q

Quotient: The answer to a division problem.

R

Ratio: A relationship between two numbers.

Reactants: The part of a chemical reaction that reacts to produce a desired end result or compound.

Reciprocals: Pairs of numbers that equal 1 when multiplied together.

Reflection: The bouncing back of a wave from a barrier or from a boundary between two media.

Refraction: The bending of a wave as it passes at an angle from one medium into another if the speed of propagation differs.

Remainder: The portion of the dividend that is not evenly divisible by the divisor.

Resistance: The property of a circuit element that impedes the flow of electricity and is measured in ohms.

Ribonucleic acid (RNA): Nucleic acid found in both the nucleus and cytoplasm of the cell; occurs in three forms: mRNA, ribosomal RNA, and tRNA.

Ribose: Sugar used in the formation of RNA.

Rough ER: Section of the endoplasmic reticulum (ER) that is covered with ribosomes; responsible for protein synthesis and membrane production.

Run-on sentence: Two or more complete sentences are written as though they were one sentence.

S

Sarcomeres: Segments of muscle cells (fibers) consisting of myofibrils.

Scalar quantity: Quantity described simply by a numeric value.

Scientific notation: The scientific system of writing numbers; a method to write very big or very small numbers easily; composed of three parts: a mathematic sign (+ or −), the significand, and the exponential, sometimes called the *logarithm.*

Sentence: A group of words that expresses a complete thought.

Sentence fragment: Incomplete sentence.

Series circuit: A circuit with only one pathway through which current can flow, so current is the same through all resistors.

Sexist language: Spoken or written styles that unnecessarily identify gender.

Significand: The base value of the number or the value of the number when all the values of ten are removed. Used in scientific notation.

Single replacement: Reactions that consist of a more active metal reacting with an ionic compound containing a less active metal to produce a new compound.

Sliding filament model: Mechanism of muscle contraction in which myosin binds to actin, and pulls it toward the center of the sarcomere.

Smooth ER: Section of the endoplasmic reticulum (ER) that lacks ribosomes; functions in detoxification and metabolism of multiple molecules.

Solute: The part of a solution that is being dissolved.

Solution: A homogeneous mixture of two or more substances.

Solvent: The part of the solution that is doing the dissolving.

Steroid: Lipid that is a component of a cell membrane; many steroids are precursors to significant hormones.

Stop codon: Sequence of bases that terminates translation during protein synthesis.

Subject: A word, phrase, or clause that names whom or what the sentence is about.

Superficial: Directional term meaning closer to or at the surface of the body.

Superior: Directional term meaning above.

Synonym: A word that means the same thing as another word.

Synthesis: A type of chemical reaction in which two elements combine to form a product. An example is the formation of potassium chloride (KCl) salt when a solution of potassium (K) combines with chloride (Cl−).

T

Terminating decimal: A decimal that is not continuous.

Textspeak: A language that is often used in text messages, emails, and other forms of electronic communication; it consists of abbreviations, slang, emoticons, and acronyms.

Thrombocytes: Platelets.

Tone: The attitude or feelings the author has about the topic.

Transcription: Process during protein synthesis in which the DNA molecule is used as a template to form mRNA.

Transfer RNA (tRNA): RNA involved in protein synthesis; transfers a specific amino acid to the ribosome and binds it to mRNA.

V

Valence electrons: Electrons in the outermost shell that are good conductors of electricity.

Variable: A letter representing an unknown quantity (e.g., x).

Vector quantity: Quantity describing the time rate of change of an object's position.

Velocity: Speed in a specific direction.

Verb: A word or phrase that is used to express an action or a state of being.

Voltage: The potential difference between two points and is measured in volts.

INDEX

Note: Page numbers followed by "b", "t", and "f" refer to boxes, tables, and figures respectively.